Clinical Diagnosis and Treatment of Adhesive Arachnoiditis

Handbook for the Medical Practitioner

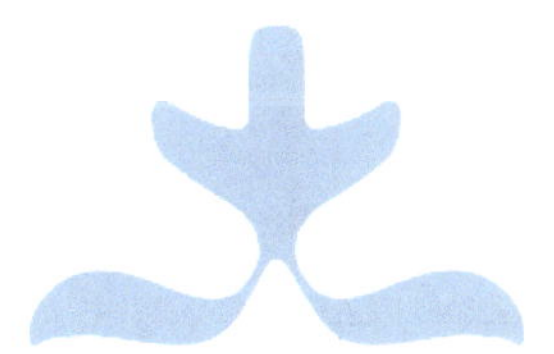

Forest Tennant, DrPH, MPH

Published by the
Tennant Foundation
West Covina, California

ISBN: 9781955934183
Library of Congress Control Number: 2022907190

Special discounts are available on quantity purchases by corporations, associations, educators, and others. For details, contact one of the parties listed below.

U.S. trade bookstores and wholesalers: Please contact
Nancy Kriskovich Tel: (406)249-2002;
or email snkriskovich@gmail.com

All proceeds from the sale of this book will go to the Medical Research and Education Projects sponsored by the
TENNANT FOUNDATION.
336 ½ S. GLENDORA AVENUE
WEST COVINA, CA 91790-3060
A 501(c)(3) Non-profit Organization

ACKNOWLEDGMENTS

Martin J. Porcelli, DO, PhD operates the Tennant Foundation Research and Education Project for Adhesive Arachnoiditis. This handbook could not have been written without his dedicated and diligent care of patients with this tragic disease.

This book could not have been researched and written without the technical and editorial assistance of Becky and Tom Marino and Nancy Kriskovich.

Advice and review of this handbook was gratefully done by Lynn Ashcraft, Donna Corley, K. Scott Guess, Pharm D, and Ryle Holder, Pharm D, Ingrid Hollis, and Martin J. Porcelli, DO, PhD.

DEDICATION

Dr. Antonio Aldrete over forty years ago mentored the author of this handbook about the tragedy and need for diagnosis and treatment of adhesive arachnoiditis.

CONTENTS

AUTHOR'S NOTES

This handbook has been written for one simple reason. Adhesive arachnoiditis (AA) can no longer be considered a rare disease. Cases can be found in every community and medical practice that encounters patients with low back pain. The incidence and prevalence of AA has markedly increased in recent years primarily due to the new ability to recognize and diagnose the disease. The new technology of contrast magnetic resonance imaging (MRI) has made it possible to definitively diagnose AA. In the past AA patients usually went undiagnosed and were inappropriately labeled with such non-descript disorders as failed back syndrome, degenerative spine, or simply low back pain. Other factors that seem to be increasing and fostering AA are intervertebral disc herniations, genetic connective tissue diseases, autoimmune collagen disorders, and excessive use of some medical procedures. We conservatively estimate that there are now at least 1.75 to 2.75 million adults in the USA who have AA.

The first major goal of this handbook is to emphasize that AA is a spinal canal inflammatory disease and not merely a pain problem. A second goal is to eradicate the long-held belief that "nothing can be done" or "there is no treatment." Although there may be no specifically labeled pharmacologic agent for AA, it, like other inflammatory diseases, responds to a variety of pharmacologic, nutrition, and physiologic measures.

My personal interest in AA was developed some 40 years ago when I encountered severe intractable pain patients who developed AA due to insoluble dyes (pantopaque, etc.) injected into the spinal canal to assist radiography. In the past five years I've retired from clinical practice to devote full-time to researching this dreadful disease. To this end, I've reviewed about 700 MRIs of documented cases and developed some simple, ambulatory protocols and recommendations that can be implemented in any medical practice. Like all medical innovations, my methods described in this handbook are a "first shot." In the 1800"s, AA was sometimes called the "Devils Disease." Those who have it today can well testify to this label. For the benefit of the patients who suffer terribly from this dreadful disease, it is my fond hope that this handbook will stimulate improvements over my initial efforts.

PART 1:

DIAGNOSIS AND PATHOGENESIS PRELUDE

These pages explain the disease of adhesive arachnoiditis and how it develops. They provide the information needed to diagnose it in every medical practice.

1. INTRODUCTION

Adhesive arachnoiditis (hereafter AA) is a lumbar-sacral spinal canal inflammatory disease in which there is a clump or group of cauda equina nerve roots that are attached by adhesions to the inside of the arachnoid-dural covering (meninges or thecal sac) of the spinal canal. [3,6,9,11,12] This disease has a typical set of symptoms, physical findings, and laboratory abnormalities. AA can be visualized and confirmed by contrast (which can separate fluid from solid tissue) magnetic resonance imaging (MRI). Non-adhesive arachnoiditis (hereafter ARC) simply means inflammation of the arachnoid layer or membrane of the spinal canal covering. ARC is essentially not visible on an MRI, and it is not a focus of this handbook. It is often a critical element in the pathogenesis of AA, however, as it often precedes or is the precursor of AA. Medical and lay literature usually refer to the singular term, arachnoiditis, when they really mean AA. Although inflammation and adhesions may adhere the spinal cord or brain to the spinal canal covering or meninges, this condition is extremely rare and due to a serious, likely terminal disease, such as an inoperable cancer, mutilating trauma, or overwhelming infection. Lumbar-sacral AA is the focus of this handbook as it is the disease that is now being seen with increasing frequency in every community and medical practice.

Currently there isn't one specific drug or surgical procedure for the treatment of AA. Also, the disease is rightfully considered to be "incurable" like diabetes, hypertension, and rheumatoid arthritis and like these diseases, it is usually controllable. In the past medical practitioners have often informed patients that the disease did not exist, and/or "nothing can be done." Today, AA is too common and easy to diagnose and treat to either deny its existence or state that "nothing can be done." This handbook provides diagnostic and treatment methods to identify causes and provide some relief, recovery, and quality of life for those afflicted with this awful disease.

2. HISTORY OF AA

The word "arachnoid" derives from the arachnoid membrane's fragile spiderweb like appearance.[2] Arachnoiditis as a distinct disease was first recognized in the mid 1800's. The common causes of arachnoiditis at that time were tuberculosis and syphilis. The famous French neurologist, Jean Martin Charcot, recorded a description of the disorder in 1869.[16] Dr. Thomas Addison, the British physician who discovered adrenal failure, published his findings on 11 autopsied patients in 1855.[1] Two of these cases had severe pain, atrophic adrenals, and calcium deposits and fluid around the arachnoid layer. The exact year the disorder was named is uncertain, but the 1873 "Comprehensive Medical Dictionary" published by J.B. Lippincott Co. included this definition: "Arachnitis: A faulty term, denoting inflammation of the arachnoid membrane."[96] The same dictionary also defined "arachnoiditis" as, "inflammation of the arachnoid membrane."

The first recorded attempt to treat arachnoiditis was probably in 1781 when Dr. John Fothergill, a famous British physician, treated a patient with severe back and sciatic pain along with other symptoms compatible with arachnoiditis.[29] Opioids failed to relieve the pain, but a mercury concoction resulted in a positive result. In 1899 the first edition of the Merck Manual listed drugs and measures for spinal meningitis with notations that the recommendations were for chronic and tubercular meningitis.[65] No less than 30 recommendations were made including opium and water baths which are still used today.

The first clinical report was published in 1909 by the esteemed British neurosurgeon, Sir Victor Horsley.[45] He operated on and described 21 patients that he believed had a spinal canal tumor with varying degrees of paraplegia. During his surgeries he found the spinal canal to be distended and to contain a considerable amount of excess fluid. Cauda equina nerve roots were edematous and "matted" together forming a mass. Inflammation encompassed all layers of the meninges. All his patients had intervertebral disc herniations that required laminectomy. Today's AA cases are similar. For example, MRIs of the spinal canal often show distention. Spinal fluid collects in the lower spinal canal, so flow is impeded. Most AA cases today have discs that protrude and press upon the spinal canal.

The second clinical description on AA was reported by S.C. Harvey in 1928.[39] He found that inflammation in the spinal canal cover affected both the arachnoid and dural layers and that cauda equina nerve roots were glued or "stuck" to the cover by adhesions. His findings are relevant because the inflammation and adhesions of AA weaken the spinal canal cover so that it loses tensile strength, dilates, and will seep or leak spinal fluid into the epidural space and tissues that surround the spinal column. This seepage can be chronic, often visualized on MRI, and cause back pain and contractures of muscle, subcutaneous tissue, and skin around the lower back. Ever since the Harvey report this disease has been called adhesive arachnoiditis (AA).

The major causes of arachnoiditis in the 1800's and early 1900's were syphilis, tuberculosis, and gonorrhea.[2] Treatment agents were developed for these infections in the 1900's so they disappeared as causes of AA. A new cause, however, originated in about 1930, when poorly soluble oil dyes were infused into the spinal canal to enhance x-ray visualization for diagnostic purposes. These x-rays were called myelograms. A small percentage of patients who received these dyes developed arachnoiditis. Magnetic Resonance Imaging (MRI) technology was developed in 1987. MRI's progressively replaced oil-based dyes and consequently, for a time, arachnoiditis seemed to almost disappear. A multiplicity of factors, however, has caused this disease to reappear in modern times.

TABLE: HISTORIC SUMMARY OF AA

1873 – Arachnoiditis defined as inflammation of the arachnoid membrane. Most common causes: syphilis and tuberculosis.

1909 – Horsley describes a dilated spinal canal, fluid stasis, nerve root "matting" (clumping) and disc protrusion.

1928 – Harvey describes adhesions and inflammation that cause cauda equina nerve roots to adhere to the spinal canal cover and produce fluid leakage through the cover. Since this report the disease has been called "Adhesive Arachnoiditis."

1900-2000 – AA recognized only as a rare disease, and the few reported cases are almost solely caused by spinal canal dyes for x-ray purposes.

1987 – MRI developed obviating most spinal canal dyes.

2000 forward – AA re-emerges in modern society. Incidence and prevalence are increasing.

3. CAUSES OF AA TODAY

In the 19th and 20th centuries AA was believed to be caused by a singular factor – infection or toxic myelogram dye. Today, AA is almost always the result of multiple factors.[4,62, 91] The only exception is a severe traumatic accident such as a vehicle accident or fall that extensively damages the bony and soft tissue elements of the lumbar-sacral spinal column. Almost all cases of AA identified in medical practice are preceded by one or more genetic or autoimmune disorders, and/or structural abnormalities of the spinal column. The most common structural abnormality that precedes AA is one or more herniated or "slipped" intervertebral discs that press upon the spinal canal and produce varying degrees of compression or stenosis.[47,52,53,103] The causes of disc herniations are many and include such lifestyle habits as obesity diabetes, smoking, lack of exercise, and excessive sitting.[26,33,81,88] Other structural abnormalities that may precede AA include scoliosis, rheumatoid spondylitis, osteoarthritis of vertebrae, spondylolisthesis, cysts in the spinal canal (Tarlov), and osteoporosis with vertebral collapse.[7,14,25,47,52,76,97]

Trauma from falls, accidents, and surgery in a person with a structural abnormality may initiate or accelerate an inflammatory response that leads to AA. Severe trauma, per se, may cause enough structural damage and inflammation to the spinal canal to cause AA.

Intervertebral discs that protrude and precede AA may occur spontaneously with no history of significant trauma or physical event such as heavy lifting. Herniated discs may be inflamed and produce elevated blood cytokines.[89,104] The inflammation in intervertebral discs may spread to the arachnoid membrane and cauda equine nerve roots leading to subsequent development of AA.[47,89,104]

Today herniated discs that precede AA are often associated with the genetic connective tissue disease, Ehlers-Danlos Syndrome (EDS), a specific autoimmune-collagen disease, or a post-infectious autoimmune-collagen disorder.[13,43,82,83] The most common autoimmune-collagen diseases we have encountered have been psoriatic arthritis and systemic lupus erythematosus. Post-infectious autoimmune-collagen disorders have primarily been due to infections with Lyme, Epstein Barr virus (EBV), or cytomegalovirus (CMV).

The major toxic chemical that entered the spinal canal and caused AA in the past century was dye (e.g., pantopaque) used in radiologic procedures. Today, chemical contaminants that may cause AA are found in epidural injection solutions used either for therapy or obstetric anesthesia.[28,31,59,69] Spinal taps may precede AA in some cases. The cause is likely that the tap allows a contaminant, including non-spinal tissue or an infectious agent, to inadvertently enter the spinal canal.

It is unclear why a rare epidural injection or spinal tap may precede or even cause AA considering that thousands of both are done with no adverse consequences.[31,35] Almost all of the AA cases in our studies, that immediately occurred following an epidural injection or spinal tap, had a herniated disc, genetic connective tissue disease, or autoimmune-collagen disorder prior to the medical procedure. Some persons with AA have had numerous epidural injections and surgical procedures. It is unclear whether these large number of procedures were necessary or caused AA, because the procedures were always done in patients who had structural abnormalities of the spine.

TABLE: CAUSES AND PRECEDING FACTORS OF AA

Structural Abnormalities of Lumbar-Sacral Spine:

- ✓ Herniated disc/spinal canal compression
- ✓ Osteoporosis with vertebral collapse
- ✓ Scoliosis
- ✓ Rheumatoid spondylitis
- ✓ Spinal canal cysts (Tarlov)
- ✓ Spondylolisthesis
- ✓ Vertebral osteoarthritis

Autoimmune-Collagen Diseases:

- ✓ Psoriatic arthritis
- ✓ Systemic lupus erythematosus

Autoimmune Collagen Disorders:

- ✓ Genetic connective tissue diseases: Ehlers-Danlos Syndromes (EDS) or Marfan Syndrome
- ✓ Post infections: Epstein Barr virus, Lyme, Cytomegalovirus

Toxic Chemical:

- ✓ Epidural injection contaminants
- ✓ Spinal tap contaminant entry

Trauma:

- ✓ Accidents
    - Automobile
    - Falls
- ✓ Surgery

4. NO LONGER A RARE DISEASE

In the past AA has been considered a rare disease.[4,51,75,87] This is no longer the case. Patients with AA are now seen in every community and medical practice that encounters persons with low back pain. There are multiple reasons for the emergence of AA in this century.

Certain lifestyle habits have increased the incidence and prevalence of intervertebral disc herniations which may precede AA. These include excessive sitting, obesity, lack of exercise, smoking, and high carbohydrate intake.[5,6,54,81] Some observers believe epidural injections and surgery have helped increase the prevalence of AA.[31,35] Genetic connective tissue and autoimmune collagen disorders have either increased or are now being recognized.[41] Some infections, particularly the Epstein Barr virus, is now recognized as a cause of spinal canal diseases.[10,38]

MRIs have made it possible to diagnose and confirm the presence of AA, when, in the past, a lack of this advanced diagnostic tool meant that cases went undiagnosed. [24,80] In summary there are multiple reasons why AA is now being recognized at a rate that can't be considered "rare". In addition each person with AA usually has multiple contributing factors that cause the disease.

Although the precise incidence (new cases) and prevalence (identified cases) are unknown, we have been able to estimate a prevalence range. Between 2000 and 2007 the total number of adults in the USA with disabling chronic back pain increased

64% from 7.8 to 12.9 million.[33] A conservative estimate is that at least 25% of persons with disabling chronic back pain have AA which translates to between 1.75 to 2.75 million adults. Several epidemiologic studies in recent years have validated that the number of persons with significant or "high impact" chronic pain numbers over 20 million people.[22,26,42,46,67,68,74,86,88] It is entirely possible that AA may be higher in prevalence than our estimate.

5. PATHOLOGIC DESCRIPTION OF AA

AA is an inflammatory disease of the lumbar-sacral spinal canal in which nerve roots of the cauda equina are adhered ("glued") to the inside of the arachnoid-dural (meninges) covering of the canal. The pathologic process that causes AA with the attachment of cauda equina nerve roots to the covering of the spinal canal occurs when one of these two tissues initially becomes inflamed, produces adhesions, and then sticks the two tissues together. An intraspinal canal mass is formed which entraps some nerve roots that innervate the lower extremities, bladder, gastrointestinal tract, and sex organs.[18,78,99] Constant pain is produced that may become severe, intractable, and disabling.[22,41,61,62,93,94] The inflammatory adhesive mass that is formed inside the spinal canal alters and impairs spinal fluid flow.[23,57,102] The lumbar-sacral spinal canal covering may be inflamed and lose its tensile strength, weaken, dilate, leak, and collect spinal fluid. The stasis of fluid collection in the bottom of the spinal canal may interfere with normal fluid flow in the upper part of the spinal canal and brain. This may lead to a variety of symptoms in the neck, upper extremities, ears, eyes, and nose.

DIAGRAM: NORMAL LATERAL VIEW OF THE CAUDA EQUINA

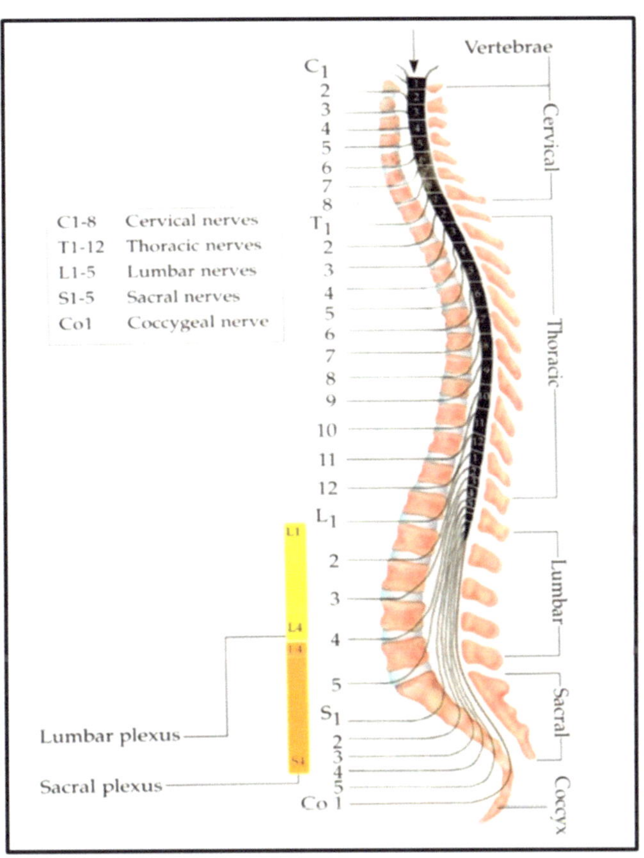

Note: The cauda equina nerve roots emanate from the lower thoracic and upper lumbar regions of the spinal cord. The nerve roots are freely suspended in spinal fluid

DIAGRAM: AA IN LUMBAR-SACRAL SPINAL CANAL

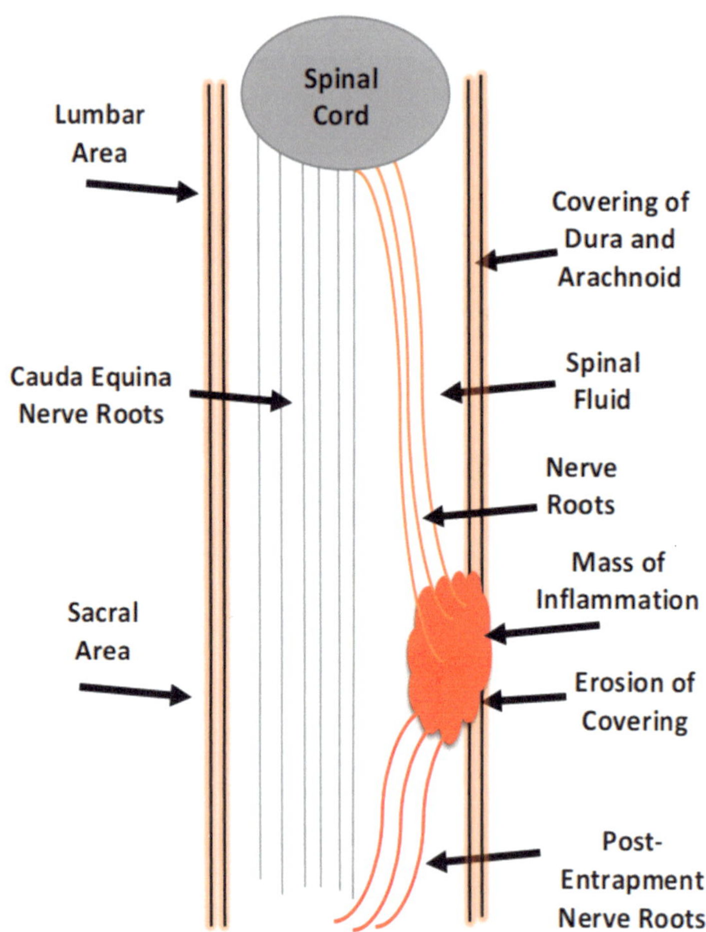

Note: Some of the cauda equina nerve roots are entrapped in a mass that is attached to the spinal canal cover. This entrapment causes severe pain and neurologic impairments of the bladder, gastrointestinal tract, sex organs, and lower extremities.

DIAGRAM: NORMAL AXIAL APPEARANCE OF THE LUMBAR-SACRAL SPINAL CANAL

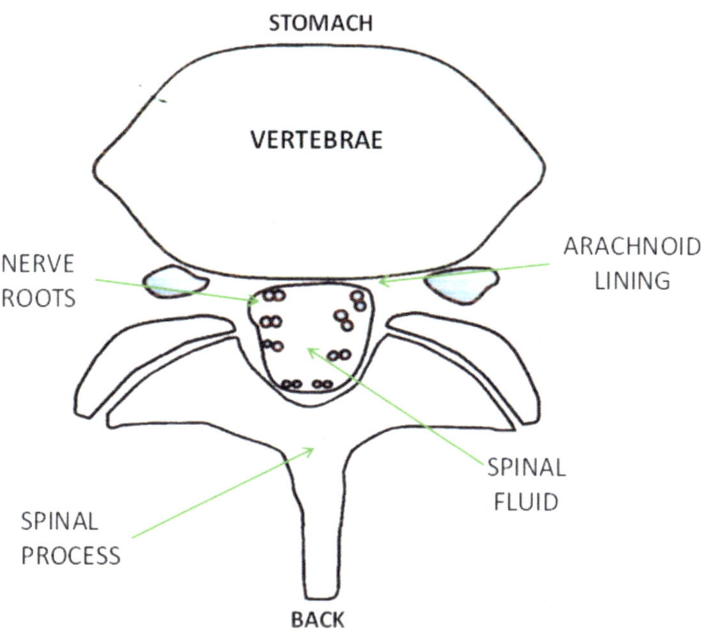

Note: The diagram here is at about the L4-L5 level. Cauda equina nerve roots number about two dozen on an MRI. They appear circular and are paired in a standard, symmetrical pattern with equal numbers on the right and left side of the spinal canal.[18,99] When nerve roots become inflamed, they appear thickened due to edema. They may be displaced and appear shifted and disorganized compared to their normal, symmetrical pattern.

The basic appearance of AA is a clump of nerve roots that is adhered by inflammatory adhesions to the inside of the spinal canal covering. Below is a diagram of a single clump in the spinal canal that is adhered to the inside of the spinal canal covering.

DIAGRAM: SINGLE NERVE ROOT CLUMP OF AA IN SPINAL CANAL

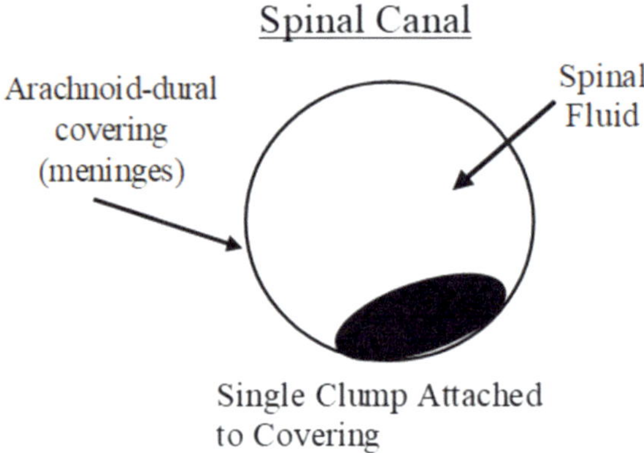

Note: The cauda equina nerve roots that are entrapped in the clump or mass cause the specific symptoms that are present in each patient. Nerve roots that are commonly entrapped include those that enervate the bladder, gastrointestinal tract, sex organs, and lower extremities.

MRI: SINGLE CLUMP OF AA IN SPINAL CANAL

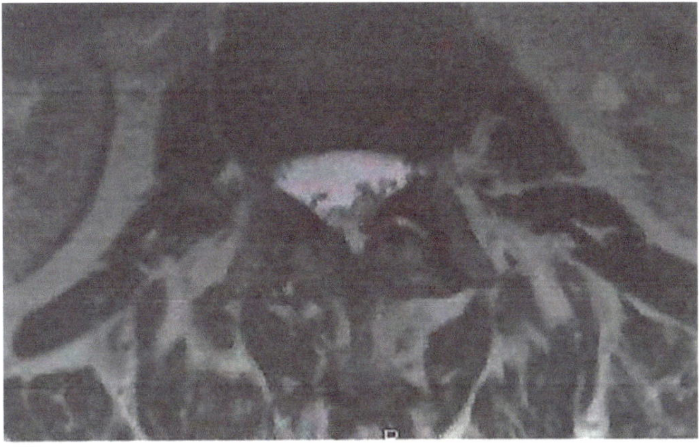

Note: MRI image of a single clump of nerve roots attached to the arachnoid-dural covering at about L4-L5.

The nerve roots have lost their circular contour and are displaced to the right. Spacing between roots cannot be visualized.

Many clinical cases of AA show multiple clumps or masses attached to the inside of the spinal canal covering on an axial contrast MRI.

DIAGRAM: MULTIPLE NERVE ROOT CLUMPS IN SPINAL CANAL

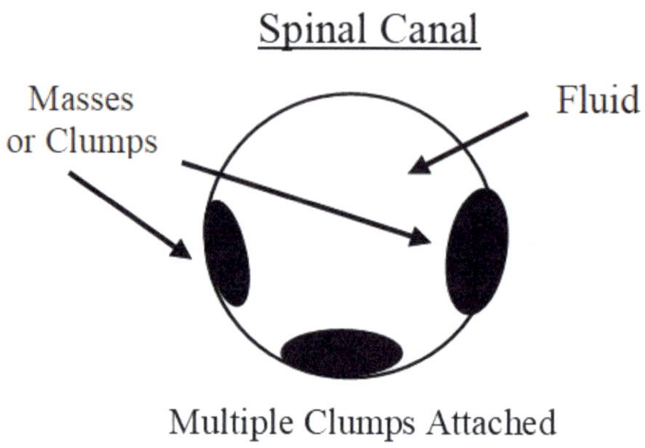

Note: Many AA patients demonstrate more than one clump of nerve roots inside the lumbar sacral spinal canal. This situation is usually associated with the most severe pain and neurologic impairments.

MRI: MULTIPLE CLUMPS OF AA IN SPINAL CANAL

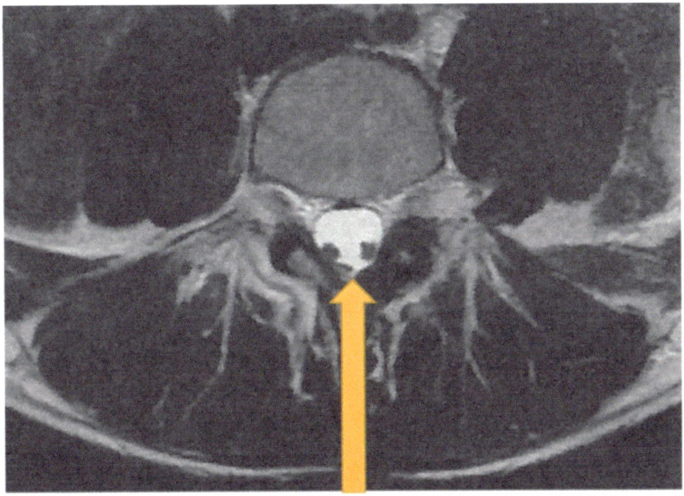

Note: Multiple nerve root clumps are adhered to the inside of the spinal canal cover. The clumps are dense as individual nerve roots cannot be identified. Tight adherence to the canal cover is sometimes called peripheralization. Dense clumps can calcify which suggests non-functional nerve roots.[85] These findings are typically found in patients who are bedbound, deteriorating and require palliative care.

MRI: NORMAL LATERAL VIEW OF LUMBAR SACRAL SPINAL CANAL

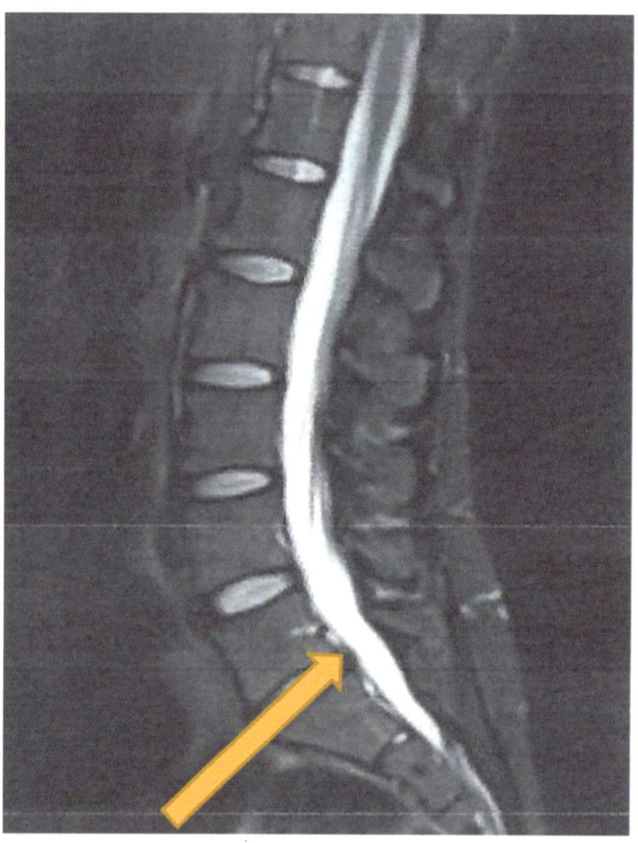

Note: Normal lateral view of the spinal canal. The white is spinal fluid. Normally a gray color inside the spinal canal represents the spinal cord or cauda equina nerve roots. A gray color may also indicate a disease process is present.

MRI: AA MASS ON LATERAL VIEW OF THE LUMBAR SACRAL SPINAL CANAL

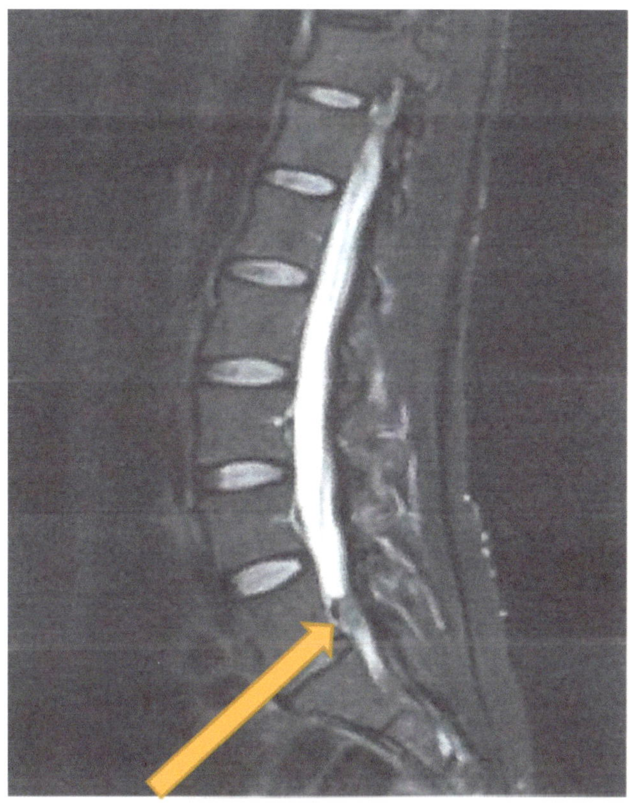

Note: Adhesive arachnoiditis is present. The arrow points to a clump of nerve roots that has resulted from inflammation and adhesions. There is adherence of the mass to the arachnoid-dural canal covering. This mass obstructs normal spinal fluid flow.

6. MAJOR SYMPTOMS OF AA

Major symptoms of AA are fairly typical. This is due to the inflamed adhesive mass of AA which is usually in close proximity to the lumbar-sacral junction. It is this location where pressure on the spinal column is maximal upon sitting and is the most common location for disc protrusion and herniation. Cauda equina nerve roots at this location enervate the bladder, gastrointestinal tract, sex organs, and nerves to the lower extremities.[18]

TABLE: COMMON SYMPTOMS OF AA

- ✓ Constant back pain
- ✓ Shooting pains into buttocks, legs, or feet
- ✓ Pain with sitting, relieved by standing or reclining
- ✓ Burning or electrical shocks in feet
- ✓ Sensation of water running or insects crawling on legs
- ✓ Blurred vision, headaches, tinnitus

A common occurrence, in addition to constant pain, is that the pain increases when sitting too long but relieved when standing or reclining. Urinary symptoms of hesitancy, dripping, nocturia, and even incontinence may occur. Gastrointestinal symptoms can vary from constipation, bloating, pain, and diarrhea. Gastroparesis may occur. Loss of sexual function is common. There are usually burning pains in the feet or buttocks and the sensation or paresthesia's of water dripping or running or insects crawling on the lower extremities is common. Nerves to the legs can also be affected and cause varying degrees of weakness, and in severe cases, paraplegia. Electromyograms, however, are usually normal. Interestingly, patients with AA frequently complain of headache, blurred vision, or tinnitus. These symptoms are believed to be due to spinal fluid flow impairment.[23,57,102] We have developed a symptom-based screening questionnaire to aid in the diagnosis of AA. It is below and can be copied to use in medical practice.

TABLE: DIAGNOSTIC SCREENING TEST FOR ADHESIVE ARACHNOIDITIS (AA)

	QUESTIONS	YES	NO
1	In addition to chronic pain, do you ever experience sharp, stabbing pains in your lower back when you twist, turn or bend?		
2	Do you ever experience bizarre skin sensations such as crawling insects or water dripping down one or both legs?		
3	Do you ever have burning, tingling, or a sensation of walking on broken glass in your feet and/or toes?		
4	Does your pain become worse while standing, sitting, and/or walking?		
5	Do you have leg weakness and/or pain that radiates down one or both legs?		
6	Do you experience any bladder dysfunction such as dribbling, or difficulty when starting or stopping urination?		
7	Do you sometimes have a headache along with blurred vision?		
8	Have you been told you have spinal discs that are protruding (bulging) into your spinal canal, scoliosis, osteoporosis, or other spine disorder?		
Note	**If a person answers yes to five or more of these questions, the diagnosis of AA should be confirmed with laboratory tests, physical examination, and a contrast MRI.**		

7. WHO GETS AA?

Patients who are encountered in medical practice have a rather standard profile. AA is predominantly a female disease with a ratio of about three or four to one over males. Patients are primarily middle-aged but may range from teenager to elderly years. The majority have had herniated discs, spine surgeries, and epidural injections. Some AA patients have had a surprising number of spine surgeries and epidural injections. These invasive procedures probably had some impact on either causation or promotion of AA. Low back pain is the major complaint encountered in medical practice. Its major characteristic is that it is worsened upon sitting.

As part of our AA research and education project we have begun collecting demographic and clinical data to develop a clinical profile of who get this tragic disease. Shown here is the clinical profile of 80 patients from across the country who have AA documented by MRI. Future studies will undoubtably refine our initial efforts, but we present the table below to help medical practitioners identify current patients in their practice who may have AA.

TABLE: CLINICAL PROFILE OF 80 MRI-DOCUMENTED CASES OF ADHESIVE ARACHNOIDITIS

	NO.
1. Females	65 – 81%
2. Males	15 – 19%
3. Age Range in Years	18 to 80
4. Mean Age ± S.D. in Years	48.9 ± 13.7
5. No. with a Predisposing Spinal Condition	61 – 76.3%
a. Herniated discs	44 – 55%
b. Spondylolisthesis	17 – 21.25%
c. Osteoporosis	6 – 7.5%
d. Spine arthritis	23 – 28.75%
e. Scoliosis	9 – 11.25%
f. Tarlov cysts	9 – 11.25%
6. No. with One or More Spinal Surgeries	43 – 53.8%
7. Total No. of Spine Surgeries in 43 Cases	91
8. Range of Surgeries in 43 Cases	1 to 8
9. No. Who Had 2 or More Spine Surgeries	22 – 27.5%
10. No. Who Had One or More Epidural Injections	69 – 86.3%
11. Total No. Epidural Injections in 69 Cases	236
12. Range of Epidural Injections in 69 Cases	1 to 20
13. No. Reported Over 8 Epidural Injections	16 – 20.0%
14. Symptoms and Complications Reported by Over 55% of Cases	
a. Pain Relief on standing	70 – 87.5%
b. Standing Too Long Causes Need to Lie Down	69 – 86.3%
c. Hurts to Lie Flat on Back	67 – 83.8%
d. Pain Always Present	66 – 82.5%
e. Shooting Pains, Tremors, or Jerking in Legs	64 – 78.8%

f.	Burning Pains in Feet	63 – 78.8%
g.	Cold Hands or Feet	58 – 72.5%
h.	Crawling of Insects on Ski	58 – 72.5%
i.	Water Dripping/Running Down Legs	53 – 66.3%
j.	Difficulties Starting Urination Or Defecation	51 – 63.8%
k.	Leg Raise Hurts Back	50 – 62.5%
l.	Blurred Vision	47 – 58.8%
m.	Pain Behind Eyes	45 – 56.3%

8. CONSEQUENCES AND COMPLICATIONS

In the 1800's AA was often known as the Devil's Disease. No wonder. AA may produce the worst pain imaginable, paralysis, bladder-bowel-stomach-sex organ dysfunction, adrenal failure, and a suffering early death.[3,12] The devastation of this disease primarily comes from the pathologic consequences of an inflammatory-adhesive spinal canal mass that entraps nerve roots. Also, the mass may impair spinal fluid flow which may lead to headaches, blurred vision, and mental dysfunction.

Deaths from AA occur from adrenal or cardiac failure, and/or overwhelming sepsis.

AA can be staged or categorized as mild, moderate, and/or severe, and catastrophic. A major goal of this handbook is to identify as many patients as possible while they are still in the mild or moderate stages. The end stage consequences and complications warrant aggressive measures to hopefully prevent their occurrence.

TABLE: SOME PATHOLOGIC CONSEQUENCES OF AA

- ✓ Intractable, constant pain
- ✓ Spinal fluid leakage
- ✓ Spinal fluid flow obstruction
- ✓ Dysfunction of gastrointestinal tract, sex organs, and bladder
- ✓ Lower extremity paralysis
- ✓ Headache
- ✓ Mental dysfunction

Since the entrapment of cauda equina nerve roots never "eases" or "takes a break," pain is constant and may bring about misery, insomnia, anorexia, a bed-bound state, and hormonal deficiencies.[94]

PICTURE: CATASTROPHIC CASE OF AA

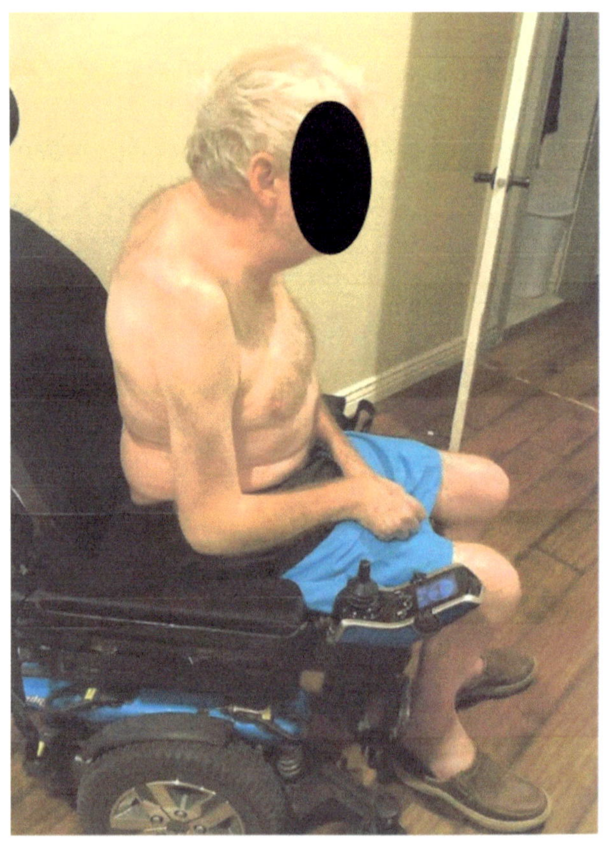

Note: Man in his mid-50's with end stage AA with leg paralysis, muscle wasting, wrist contractures and dementia. He is bed bound unless in a wheelchair. Patient has AA and an autoimmune-collagen disorder.

9. PHYSICAL EXAMINATION

There is no single, specific physical finding that identifies the person with AA. All persons with AA will, however, demonstrate a rather typical set of physical abnormalities. Since most persons with AA have protruding discs, physical findings that are usually found with disc disease will be present. For example, pain will usually be elicited with straight leg raising. The general appearance of back musculature and posture may be greatly altered due to pain, surgeries, and spinal fluid leakage. Most AA patients will splint or bend to one-side to minimize severe pain. Another factor is chronic spinal fluid seepage through a damaged spinal canal covering. Spinal fluid is an irritant to tissues outside the spinal canal, and it may cause contractures of tissue. Consequently, some severe AA cases may not be able to fully extend their upper extremities. This finding is believed to be a result of long-standing spinal fluid seepage with subsequent inflammation and contractures of the paraspinal muscles. Skin indentations are common due to contracture of subcutaneous tissues. Indentations may be the result of surgery, but some appear independent of surgical incisions. Although non-specific and variable between patients, there are almost always some physical abnormalities present in the lower extremities. Weakness and varying degrees of paraplegia may be present. Some patients cannot raise their knees and maintain balance while standing. Gait may be wide-based or unsteady. One or more reflexes are usually absent. Vibratory and touch sensations may be diminished.

Pressure along the spine may or may not elicit pain or discomfort, because the inflammatory-adhesive mass in the inside of the spinal canal is two to four inches below the skin surface. When pain can be elicited on pressure along the spinal column it probably represents chronic spinal fluid seepage through the spinal canal covering into soft tissues around the spinal column. Alternatively, some encroachment ("pinched") of nerve roots in or around foraminal exits may elicit pain on pressure. Impairments of strength, mobility, and flexibility of both arms and legs may occur in AA patients.

TABLE: SUMMARY OF TYPICAL PHYSICAL ABNORMALITIES

- ✓ Weak lower extremities
- ✓ Diminished reflexes
- ✓ Distorted back anatomy
- ✓ Muscular contractures and indentations of back
- ✓ Diminished vibratory-positional sensation
- ✓ Pain on straight leg raising
- ✓ Pain on spinal process pressure
- ✓ Diminished upper extremity extension
- ✓ Muscle wasting-late stages
- ✓ Foot drop

Note: There is no single, diagnostic physical sign of AA, but multiple, non-specific signs will be present.

PICTURE: CASE OF PSORIATIC ARTHRITIS AND AA

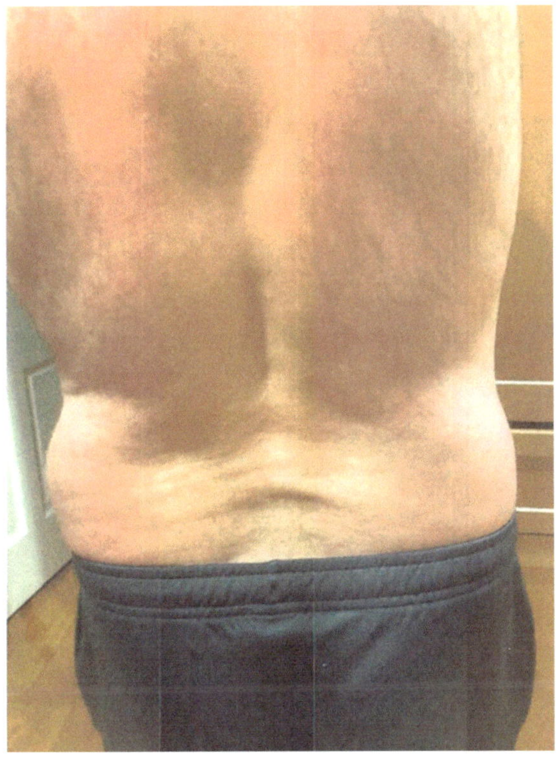

Note: Patient has not had surgery. There is midline indentation and skin-muscle contractures. He splints to the left as indicated by a skin crease. Medical practitioners should suspect AA if a patient presents with multiple anatomical abnormalities of the lower back.

PICTURE: BACK OF AA PATIENT

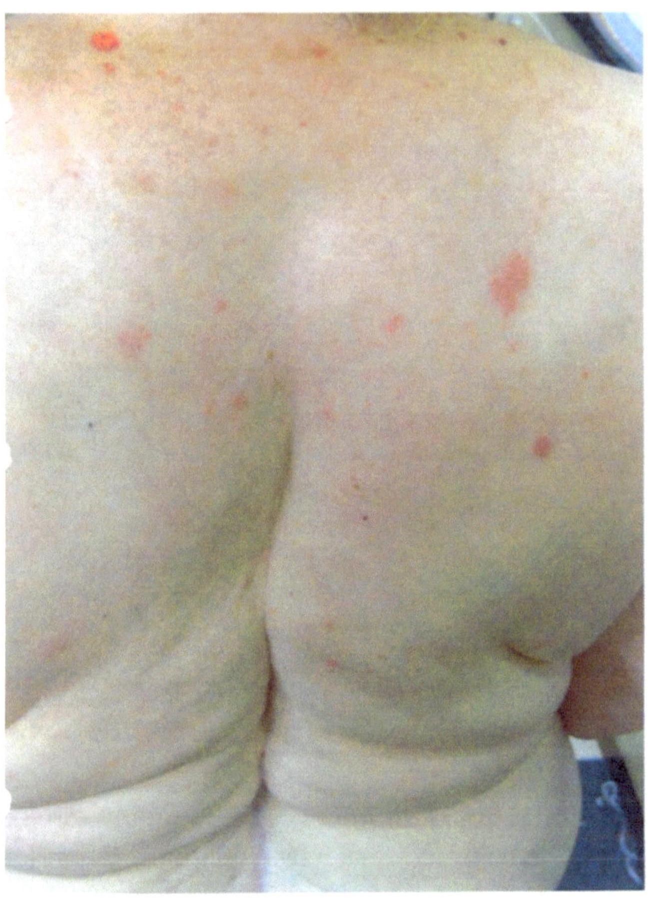

Note: There is distortion of muscle structure, skin contractures, and midline indentations. Patient is post-surgical (laminectomy). AA was confirmed in this patient by contrast MRI of the lumbar-sacral spine.

PICTURE: BACK OF AA PATIENT

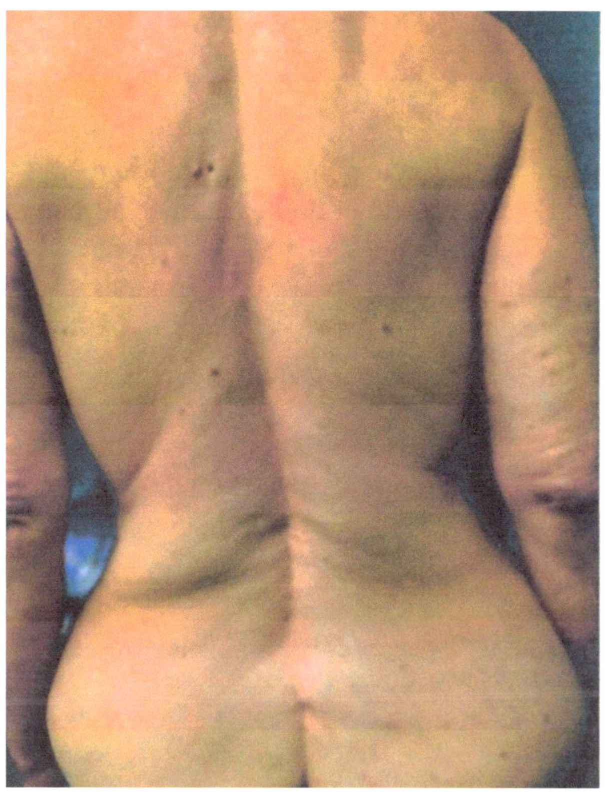

Note: There is distorted muscle structure, skin contractures, and midline indentations. Patient is post-surgical (lumbar fusion). She splints to the left as indicated by skin crease. Severe AA usually develops over a considerable time period, and it may be reflected by multiple anatomic abnormalities of the back.

10. LABORATORY TESTS

AA is a spinal canal inflammatory disease, so inflammatory marker testing is advisable, if financially feasible.[9] It is also commonly associated with or the result of an autoimmune collagen disorder. Patients should, therefore, have an erythrocyte sedimentation rate (ESR), C-reactive protein (CRP), and a cytokine panel that contains multiple leukotrienes and tumor necrosis factor.[56,64,100]

The presence of elevated inflammatory markers indicates that an inflammatory process is in the body but not necessarily in the spinal canal.[70] The absence of elevated inflammatory markers does not mean, however, that inflammation is extinguished, controlled, or won't return. We have tracked inflammation makers in AA patients over time.[9] As with rheumatoid arthritis, the markers may "wax and wane" with exacerbations and remissions.

The hormones cortisol, pregnenolone, dehydroepiandrosterone (DHEA), and testosterone among others may be lowered due to the extreme stress and pain of AA.[93] Glucose may be elevated due to dietary habits and need to be controlled as prediabetes or diabetes may retard healing, enhance pain, and predispose to disc herniation. The white blood cell (WBC) count may also be elevated due to chronic inflammation and/or autoimmunity. Antinuclear autoantibody (ANA) titers may periodically elevate. Most AA patients show extremely high Epstein Barr virus antibody (EBV) levels.[10,38] A lesser number of AA patients have elevated cytomegalovirus or Lyme titers.

There is the mistaken view that electromyograms (EMG) always show abnormalities in AA. This is seldom the case. EMG testing no longer has a place in the diagnosis of AA, as it can be misleading.

In summary, AA does not have a specific, diagnostic laboratory test. It does, however, often have elevation of inflammatory markers, white blood cell count, glucose, antinuclear autoantibody titer, and EBV antibody levels. Some hormone levels will lower below normal due to excess stress and pain.

TABLE: SUMMARY OF LABORATORY TESTING

- ✓ Inflammatory markers have periods of elevation and normalcy
- ✓ Multiple hormones may be diminished
- ✓ The following are often elevated:
  - White blood cell count
  - Glucose
  - Antinuclear autoantibody titer
  - Epstein Barr virus antibodies

Note: Although there is no specific diagnostic laboratory test for AA, a number of tests help to establish a diagnosis, identify the causation factors of AA, and guide treatment.

11. CATEGORIES OF SEVERITY

AA, like most chronic diseases, can be categorized by severity. There are four categories or stages: mild, moderate, severe, and catastrophic. As AA is becoming more recognized, treatment is thankfully being started at the mild and moderate stages, so the disease will hopefully not progress to the severe and catastrophic stages. Unfortunately, and tragically, the severe and catastrophic stages are associated with disabling pain and multiple neurologic impairments that may include paraplegia, mental impairments, incontinence, and autoimmunity. Patients with AA who are newly identified and who are in the severe and catastrophic stages have, in the main, never had adequate treatment directed at spinal canal inflammation and neurogenesis.

MRI findings may not necessarily correlate with clinical severity and impairments.[44, 71] Most persons in the severe and catastrophic stages, however, show dense, scarred nerve root masses within the spinal canal. The spinal canal itself is usually dilated due to scarring and loss of tensile strength in the canal covering. Calcification may develop in the scarred masses.[85]

Categorization or staging of AA has some practical value in treatment approach. Those persons in the mild and moderate categories seem to greatly benefit from the medical protocol outlined in a later chapter in this handbook. The protocol includes inflammation suppression and neurogenic treatment. Those persons in the severe or catastrophic stages may not respond well to anti-inflammatory and neurogenic treatment attempts as they have sustained permanent damage to cauda equina nerve roots. Symptoms in these stages may not be reversible so these patients primarily need intractable pain and palliative care.

TABLE: CATEGORIZATION AND STAGING OF AA

Stage One-Mild

- ✓ Extremities: full range of motion, strength, extension
- ✓ No urinary or central* symptoms
- ✓ Normal ambulation
- ✓ Intermittent pain. Non-opioid management is sufficient.

Stage Two-Moderate

- ✓ Extremities: full range of motion, strength, extension
- ✓ Some urinary, gastrointestinal tract, and/or central symptoms
- ✓ Normal ambulation
- ✓ Constant pain, but manageable without opioids

Stage Three-Severe

- ✓ Extremities: some deficiency in range of motion, strength, or extension
- ✓ Has significant urinary, gastrointestinal tract, and/or central symptoms
- ✓ Ambulates with assistance
- ✓ Severe constant pain that requires opioids

Stage Four-Catastrophic

- ✓ Extremities: significant deficiencies in range of motion, strength, or extension
- ✓ Significant urinary, gastrointestinal tract, or central symptoms
- ✓ Bed bound some of each day
- ✓ Ambulation requires assistance
- ✓ Severe intractable pain that requires palliative care and daily opioids

Notes on Interpretation

- ✓ Central refers to headaches, eye/ear/nasal symptoms such as blurred vision, tinnitus, vertigo, or nasal dripping
- ✓ Ambulation assistance means cane, walker, or wheelchair
- ✓ MRI findings do not necessarily correlate with staging although the severe and catastrophic categories usually show one or more of these findings: dense scarring of nerve root clumps, multiple clumps, lower spinal canal distension ("empty sac"), peripheralization, and/or calcification.[44,71]

Note: Categories can overlap. Mild and moderate categories have the best potential for recovery which is motivation to diagnose AA and begin early treatment.

MRI: SEVERE CASE OF AA

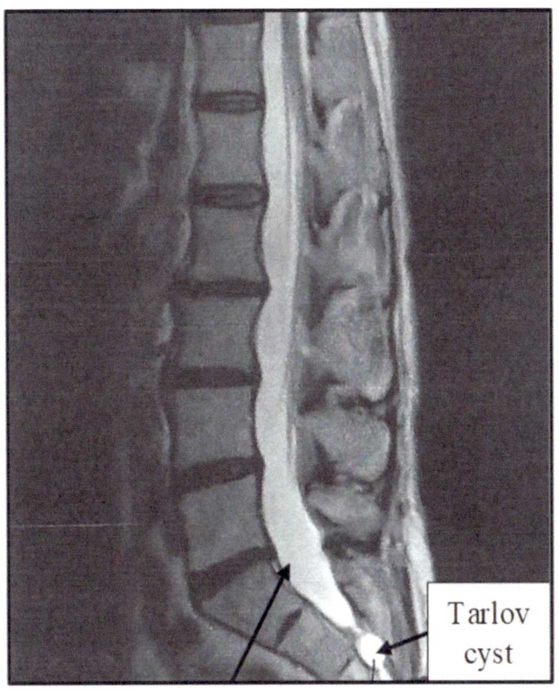

Note: This severe patient reveals a dilated or "empty sac." Multiple discs press upon the spinal canal. A cyst is in the spinal canal. This patient must walk with a walker, has intermittent gastroparesis, severe constipation, and incontinence. Pain is severe, constant, and requires opioids for control.

MRI: CATASTROPHIC CASE OF AA

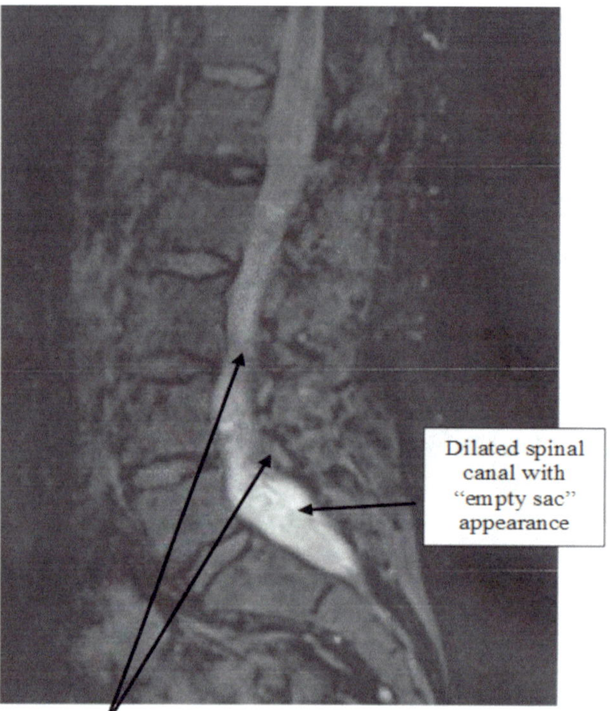

Note: This catastrophic patient shows multiple scarred AA masses on her MRI. Dilation of the lower spinal canal is present. Spinal fluid has collected in the lower canal. Patient is essentially bed bound, requires periodic catheterization to urinate, has lapses of memory, and requires a wheelchair to ambulate. Palliative, end-of-life care with daily opioids is required for relief and quality of life.

12. CRITERIA FOR A DIAGNOSIS OF AA

A diagnosis of AA requires some findings in these three categories: (1) typical symptoms of and/or abnormal laboratory tests, (2) presence of some physical abnormalities, and (3) MRI confirmation.

Although the AA patient may have numerous consequences, complications, and symptoms, two cardinal symptoms stand out. One is constant ("24/7") pain and the other is pain relief by standing or reclining. AA is a spinal canal inflammatory, nerve root entrapment disease. The entrapment is present all hours of the day and night so pain is constant although severity may vary at times from mild to severe. Standing or reclining relieves pain since the AA inflammatory, adhesive mass that entraps cauda equina nerve roots is usually located near the lumbar-sacral vertebral junction which is the major pressure impact area when one is sitting. Most AA patients cannot, therefore, sit very long. Another tell-tale symptom is some bladder/urinary dysfunction that may be hesitancy, urgency, or dripping/incontinence. Total urinary shutdown that requires catheterization may occur in severe or catastrophic cases. There are about two dozen nerve connections between the bladder and the cauda equina nerve roots. Consequently, some bladder dysfunction is almost always present even in moderate cases.

Although there is no specific laboratory test for AA, testing will usually show some abnormalities. Of particular note is that some cytokines will reflect the presence of inflammation when the ESR and CRP may be normal. Antinuclear (ANA) autoantibody is often abnormal. EBV antibody levels are usually quite high.

As stated in a previous chapter, there is no specific neurologic, physical finding that is diagnostic of AA. All AA patients will, however, have some non-specific physical findings due to nerve root entrapment inside the spinal canal. Such common findings are leg weakness and pain on straight leg raising. Many will show anatomic, structural abnormalities of muscle groups and skin on the back.

Electromyograms (EMG) are seldom abnormal because the disease of AA is inside the spinal canal. EMG should no longer be used to diagnose AA.

Once some typical symptoms, laboratory abnormalities and physical abnormalities have been identified, the diagnosis of AA is confirmed by finding specific signs on a contrast MRI. The most specific MRI finding that confirms AA is a nerve root clump(s) that has become adhered ("glued") to the inner wall of the arachnoid-dural covering of the spinal canal. A distended lumbar sacral spinal canal is also a specific sign of AA.

It is emphasized that a diagnosis of AA require findings in all these categories. This is seldom a difficult or questionable process since AA is a serious, demonstrable, pathologic disease.

TABLE: DIAGNOSTIC CRITERIA FOR AA

Category	Common Findings
Symptoms and laboratory abnormalities	✓ Constant pain ✓ Pain relief on standing or reclining ✓ Bladder dysfunction ✓ Elevated inflammatory markers
Physical Findings	✓ Leg weakness ✓ Decreased reflexes ✓ Pain on straight leg raising ✓ Anatomic distortion of the back
MRI	✓ Nerve root clumps adhered to arachnoid-dural covering of the spinal canal ✓ Dilated spinal canal

Note: A diagnosis of AA requires a finding in all these categories.

13. PROCESS AND TIMEFRAME FOR DEVELOPMENT

AA is caused by multiple factors with the exception of severe trauma such as a vehicle accident or fall. The most common preceding condition of AA is inflamed intervertebral discs that protrude and press upon the spinal canal covering. The time frame to develop AA following a protruding disc, an infection, or autoimmune disease may range from months to years. In contrast, we have been able to determine a general time frame from an arachnoid-dural puncture or epidural injection to the presence of AA on contrast MRI. AA will not show on a contrast MRI for at least 4 to 8 weeks after an arachnoid-dural puncture or epidural injection. To develop AA there must first be inflammation in either the cauda equina nerve roots or arachnoid-dural covering of the spinal canal. The original inflammation must fester, spread, and develop adhesions that glue the nerve roots to the canal cover. Prior to the development of an MRI that shows a definite clump or mass of nerve roots attached to the covering, a contrast MRI may show some non-specific findings of normal nerve root enlargement, loss of circular contour, and/or asymmetry of the nerve root pattern. To hopefully prevent the development of AA, emergency treatment, which is described later in this handbook, should be started when symptoms of AA begin because an MRI may not show AA for several weeks.

DIAGRAM: AA DEVELOPMENTAL PROCESS FOLLOWING DURAL PUNCTURE OR EPIDURAL INJECTION

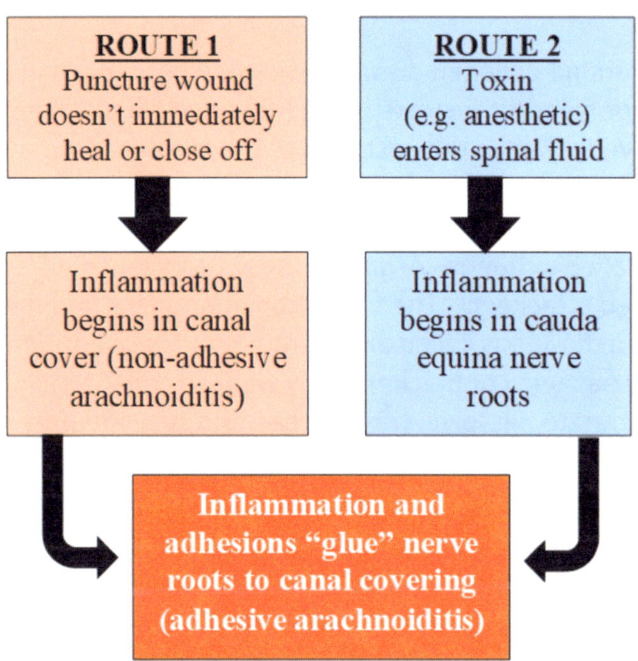

Note: The above process will usually require a minimum of four to six weeks.

14. AUTOIMMUNE COLLAGEN DISORDERS MAY CAUSE AA

Autoimmune-collagen disorders seem to be increasing in the population and/or they are being identified today when they were overlooked in the past. [48,100,105] These disorders may cause AA, and they now may, in fact, be the most common underlying cause of AA. These disorders produce small particles in the blood called antigens. Arguably these particles could be called "collagen attackers." The formation of antigens and their attack on tissues is called autoimmunity. These antigens literally eat away or biochemically weaken collagen allowing it to deteriorate, dissolve, fray, or tear, and subsequently produce inflammation, adhesions, and scarring of tissues including neural tissue. Intervertebral discs, cauda equina nerve roots, and the arachnoid-dural covering of the spinal canal are loaded with collagen that holds these tissues together. Antigens may, therefore, go after these spinal canal tissues, cause collagen to deteriorate, and lead to the development of AA. The patient may not have any awareness that they have an autoimmune condition, and their first complaint to a medical practitioner is solely related to back pain or a slipped disc.

Autoimmune disorders that may cause AA can emanate from one of three sources. One is genetic connective tissue diseases. The most common are EDS or Marfan Syndrome. A second are diseases that have long been identified as autoimmune-collagen diseases. The best known is rheumatoid arthritis. We have most frequently encountered psoriatic arthritis, rheumatoid spondylitis, and systemic lupus erythematosus in

AA patients. The third source is post-infectious. As this handbook is being written considerable research and investigation is attempting to better understand post-infectious autoimmunity. In AA patients, we have found that these three infections may develop a post-infection autoimmune-collagen disorder that contribute to the development of AA: Lyme, EBV, and cytomegalovirus (CMV). EBV is known to cause multiple sclerosis, and its post infectious autoimmunity appears to be a significant, causative factor in many AA patients.[10]

Although our data collection project was not complete at the time this Handbook was written, over 75% of our AA cases have extremely high levels of EBV antibodies. These cases have other causative factors such as trauma, structural spine abnormalities, herniated discs, and genetic connective tissue diseases which suggest that AA may result from multiple causative factors.

Many persons with AA do not know they have an autoimmune-collagen disease and believe that a spinal puncture, epidural injection, surgery, or accident to be the sole cause of their AA. It is likely that the collagen matrix in their intervertebral discs, cauda equina, or arachnoid-dural spinal canal covering was defective prior to the medical procedure or trauma. It is still unclear, but it appears to us that the combination of a medical procedures or trauma and autoimmune-collagen disease is a major cause of AA.

TABLE: THREE CATEGORIES OF AUTOIMMUNE-COLLAGEN DISORDERS THAT MAY CAUSE AA

Genetic Connective Tissue Disease
Ehlers-Danlos Syndrome (EDS)
Marfan Syndrome
Autoimmune-Collagen Disease
Psoriatic Arthritis
Systemic Lupus Erythematosus
Rheumatoid Spondylitis
Post-Infection
Lyme
Epstein Barr Virus
Cytomegalovirus

Note: Patients with AA tend to have an autoimmune collagen disorder plus other causation factors such as a spine structure abnormality or trauma.

DIAGRAM: THE AUTOIMMUNE-COLLAGEN DISORDER SEQUENCE

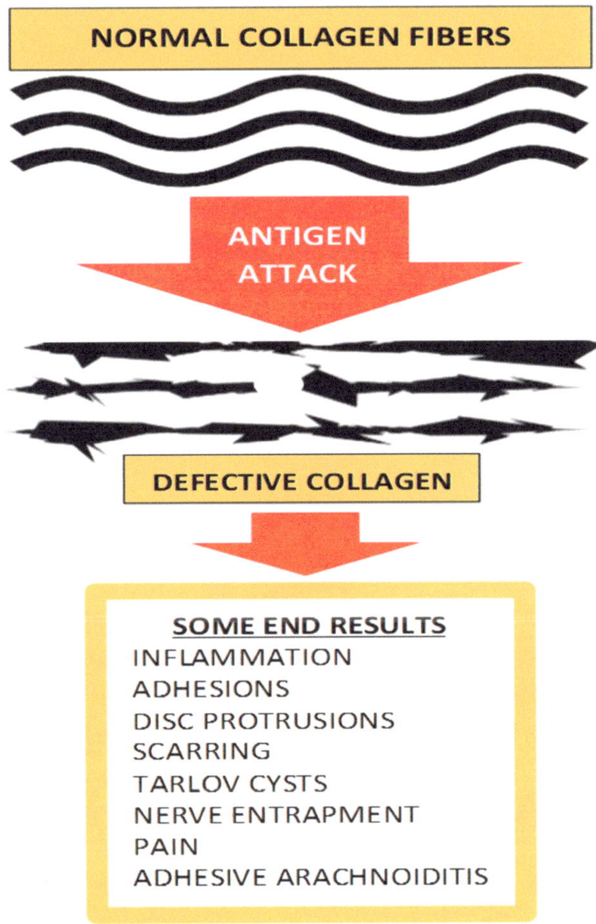

Note: The above diagram shows how an autoimmune-collagen disorder may contribute to the development of AA.

15. AUTOIMMUNE-COLLAGEN CONDITIONS OFTEN PRECEDE AA

The preceding chapter explains how an autoimmune collagen disorder may be an underlying cause of AA. Many persons with AA have common autoimmune conditions that precede or accompany AA. This chapter calls attention to some of the various clinical conditions that are now recognized as being a result of autoimmunity. Medical practitioners should now consider AA to also be the result of an autoimmune condition. A list of autoimmune conditions are listed here which may precede or accompany AA.[48,64,105] It is now incumbent upon a medical practitioner to suspect the presence of autoimmunity and the prospect that AA will or has already developed in patients who have one or more of these conditions.

Persons with a genetic connective tissue-collagen disease such as EDS or Marfan syndrome have weak immune systems. They commonly and easily acquire viral infections, particularly EBV. Persons with a post-infection autoimmune-collagen disorder may be more likely to develop AA following an epidural injection, spinal tap, surgery, or trauma.[48,64,105]

Dr. Alvin F. Coburn first coined the term "collagen disease" in 1932. He discovered that streptococcal pharyngitis (e.g., strep throat) can cause an autoimmune response that damages the collagen in the heart. The heart condition became known as rheumatic fever and rheumatic heart disease as valves would collapse due to collagen weakness. Dr. Coburn is memorialized for determining that an infectious agent can produce an autoimmune process that damages collagen. Some infections of modern times including Lyme, EBV, and CMV can produce autoimmunity as did the streptococcus prior to its control by antibiotics.

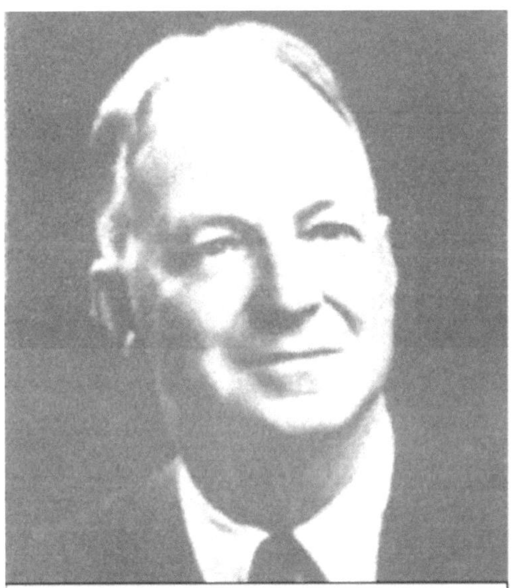

Alvin F. Coburn, 1899-1975
Discovered that an infection may cause autoimmunity and a collagen disease.

TABLE: SOME COMMON AUTOIMMUNE COLLAGEN CONDITIONS ASSOCIATED WITH AA

1	Arthritis
2	Burning mouth or feet
3	Carpal tunnel
4	Chiari conditions
5	Cold hands – Raynaud's
6	Dry eyes (Sjogren's)
7	Dysautonomia (unstable BP)
8	Fibromyalgia
9	Food-medicine sensitivities
10	Hashimoto's-thyroiditis
11	Herniated/slipped discs
12	Herpes cold sores
13	Herpes genitalia
14	Intraspinal canal fluid filled cysts (syrinx)
15	Irritable bowel
16	Mast cell activation
17	Migraine
18	Neuropathy
19	Psoriasis
20	Shingles
21	Spinal fluid leaks
22	Tarlov Cysts
23	Temporal mandibular joint (TMJ)
24	Urticaria (hives)

Note: The table here lists several well-known autoimmune manifestations. Any patient who has back pain and one or more of these autoimmune conditions should be suspected of having AA.

16. POST-INFECTION AUTOIMMUNE-COLLAGEN DISORDERS AND AA

Recent laboratory testing has revealed that the majority of patients with AA have very high antibody levels of EBV and some have high cytomegalovirus or Lyme titers.

EBV has long been known to cause autoimmune complications. For example, the author of this handbook described glomerulonephritis (kidney) with EBV in 1969, some 53 years ago.[95] Recently EBV has been shown to cause multiple sclerosis (MS) as well as certain cancers.[10] We now realize that EBV may either cause or contribute to AA as well as MS.

Although almost everyone gets infected with EBV during their lifetime, some persons develop a large number of EBV antigens that literally attack and "eat away" or otherwise cause collagen to deteriorate and weaken. If the body creates large numbers of antigens, large numbers of antibodies are simultaneously made to hopefully counter them. Anything that boosts or helps a disorder to develop, is called a "co-factor." In the case of EBV and AA, the "co-factors" or "co-partners" may include EDS, autoimmune diseases such as psoriatic arthritis, Lyme disease, and possibly some other viruses like cytomegalovirus, coxsackie, and covid. EBV "collagen eating" antigens like to attack tissues around the spine since they contain a lot of collagen. This includes intervertebral discs, cauda equina nerve roots, and the arachnoid-dural covering of the spinal canal. If collagen is weak or absent in spinal tissues, discs may slip, inflammation may form, fluid leaks, and Tarlov cysts may develop.

All persons with confirmed or suspected AA should be considered for testing of EBV, CMV, and Lyme. They should be screened for the presence of known autoimmune-collagen disorder manifestations, which are listed here. At the time this handbook is being written, there is no specific treatment recommendation for persons with AA who have high EBV antibody levels. Special treatment recommendations may come in the near future as clinical investigators are experimenting with a variety of anti-inflammatory-autoimmune and antiviral therapies to possibly suppress EBV and its attendant complications. Early reports to our AA research and education project suggest that anti-viral and low dose, corticosteroid therapy may have merit.

DIAGRAM: EBV DEVELOPMENT OF AA

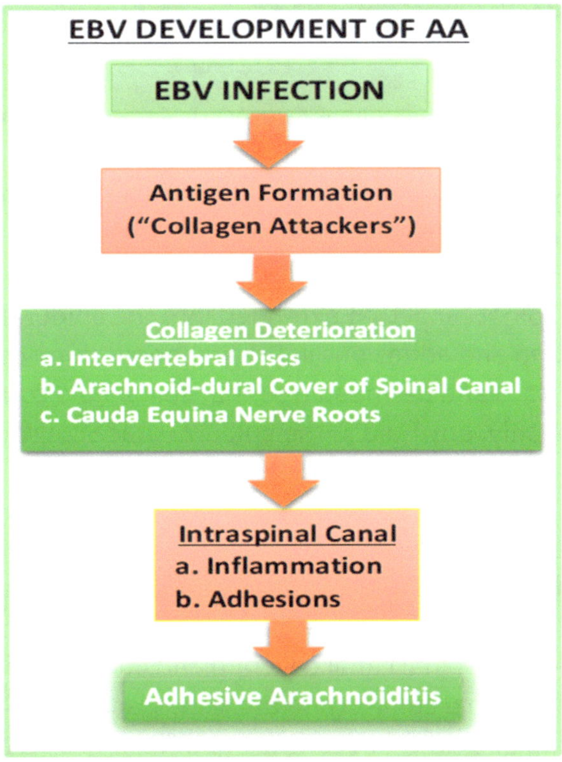

Note: EBV now appears to be a major contributing factor in many, if not most, cases of AA. The above schemata may simultaneously exist with other factors that contribute to AA such as EDS, trauma, or structural spine abnormalities.

17. SPINAL FLUID LEAKS CAUSED BY AA

In 1927, Dr. Byron Stookey, a New York neurosurgeon, reviewed all reported cases of AA.[87] His major finding was that adhesions which originate in the arachnoid layer of the spinal canal covering may also involve the dural layer.[87] This process also involved the cauda equina nerve roots and developed a mass inside the spinal canal that extended into the epidural space. Inflammation and adhesions in the arachnoid-dural covering made it porous and permeable so that spinal fluid could leak out and, conversely, any fluid in the epidural space could enter the spinal canal.

After reviewing over 700 MRIs from persons with AA, we have concluded that at least half of the persons with AA have had some chronic "seepage" or "leakage" of spinal fluid through the arachnoid-dural spinal canal covering and into the soft tissues between the spinal column and the skin. Usually the "seepage" is slow ("drip at a time") in contrast to a "leak" ("a steady stream"). One can probably have a cross between a leak and seepage.

Spinal fluid is an acidic irritant to ligaments, muscles, and fascia which are outside the spinal canal. The body attempts to push leaked spinal fluid to the skin so it can evaporate into the air. Spinal fluid that leaks into muscles and other tissues will cause inflammation and severe pain. Chronic leakage can cause muscles, tendons, subcutaneous tissue, and skin to scar and contract. In this case a person with AA may find that they can't fully extend their arms or legs or stand up straight. Pictures of some AA patients with anatomic distortion of the back with contractures are in a previous chapter of this handbook. Pain on pressure to the lower back musculature suggests active leakage with subsequent inflammation.

PICTURE: SPINAL FLUID LEAKAGE IN AA

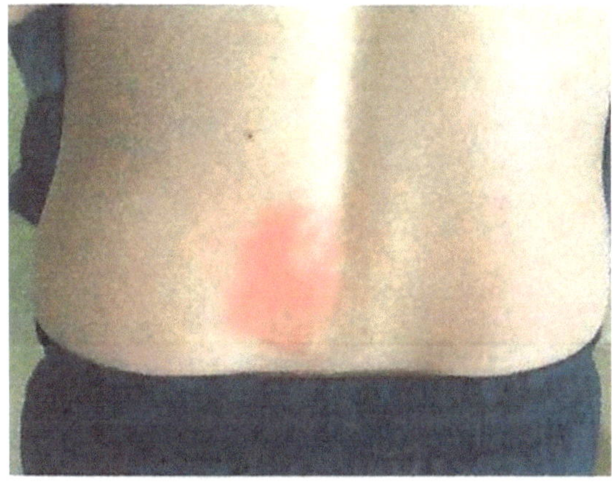

Note: The reddish spot pictured here is spinal fluid that has leaked from the spinal canal and migrated to the surface of the skin.

DIAGRAM: WHY SPINAL FLUID LEAKS IN AA

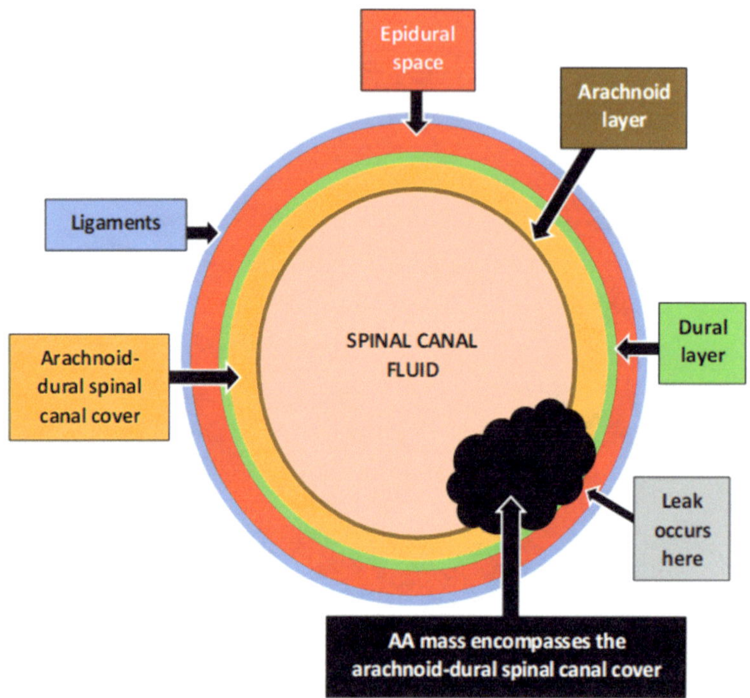

Note: This diagram shows an AA mass that encompasses the entire spinal canal covering making it porous so fluid can leave and irritate tissues outside the spinal canal. The actual size of the spinal canal is about the circumference of one's index finger.

MRI: SPINAL FLUID LEAKAGE IN AA

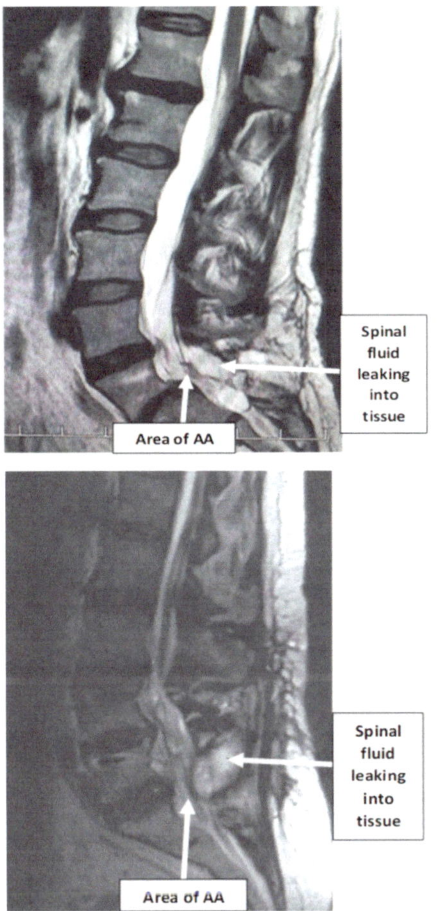

Note: Pictured here are MRI images showing spinal fluid leaks around the area of AA. Severe pain occurs with this leakage, since spinal fluid is an irritant to tissue, outside the canal.

18. CAUSES OF PREMATURE DEATH IN AA PATIENTS

Historical reports and recent clinical observations have determined that the apparent causes of a premature death in persons with AA are adrenal failure, cardiac arrest, and/or overwhelming infection or sepsis.

Persons who prematurely die with AA usually develop severe intractable pain, malnutrition, and impaired immunity. The final cause of death may therefore be an overwhelming infection. The stress and pain of AA may overwhelm the pituitary-adrenal axis so that the adrenal gland fails.[93] Interestingly, Dr. Addison described and researched adrenal failure which carries his name "Addison's' Disease." He published autopsy results on eleven patients in 1855.[1] Two of his cases had history and symptom profiles typical of AA. Post-mortems investigation showed anatomical evidence of adrenal atrophy and calcification of the arachnoid membrane.

Unfortunately, there are some persons with AA who are now being identified in medical practice who have had essentially no previous treatment that would suppress inflammation or regenerate damaged tissues. At best, they may have only received some symptomatic pain treatment. These patients may be far along in the deterioration process and be staged and categorized as severe or catastrophic. They are at risk of premature death.

Cardiac arrest may occur if an acute pain flare is so severe that the heart goes into a fatal arrythmia. Arguably the pain of AA may exceed that of any other pain including cancer bone pain. There is simply nothing more painful then nerve roots entrapped in an inflammatory, adhesive mass inside the spinal canal. Pain flares that emanate from this condition may elevate blood pressure, pulse rate, and cardiac demand so much that death may occur. In summary, the risks of premature death in AA patients is so great that aggressive anti-inflammatory, neurodegenerative, and pain control treatments are essential.

PART 2:

TREATMENT AND CARE PRELUDE

These pages provide recommendations and suggestions for care and treatment of adhesive arachnoiditis by community-based, medical practitioners. The disease is now so common that treatment cannot be totally delegated to referral centers or specialists.

19. TREATMENT NO LONGER HOPELESS

Until recently the view of AA has been that it is a "hopeless" disease, and "nothing can be done for it." These old beliefs are no longer true. New understanding of the disease and clinical experience show that AA is usually a controllable disease and treatment can provide some relief and recovery.

The major breakthrough has been the clarification that AA is an inflammatory disease inside a closed space, the spinal canal. It is very analogous to rheumatoid arthritis (RA), an inflammatory disease in a closed space, a joint. Fortunately, RA now has biologic pharmaceuticals that specifically target this disease. As of yet, AA does not have any specific biologic agent that targets it. Consequently, AA is treated in a similar fashion to how RA was treated prior to development of biologics.[34] This includes corticosteroids, anti-inflammatories, specific physical exercises, and nutritional measures.

TABLE: SIMILARITIES BETWEEN RA AND AA

Similarities Between RA and AA	RA	AA
Controllable-not curable	Y	Y
Inflammatory disorder	Y	Y
Causes tissue destruction	Y	Y
Responds to corticosteroids	Y	Y
Responds to specific anti-inflammatories	Y	Y
Inflammation may stop or "burn out"	Y	Y
Inflammation has remissions and exacerbations	Y	Y

Note: The similarities between RA and AA are interesting and summarized in the above table. They are, however, different in that the corticosteroids and anti-inflammatory agents that work in AA may not work in RA and vice versa.

20. GOALS OF DIAGNOSIS AND TREATMENT

Like most other chronic diseases, the earlier the diagnosis and start of treatment in the course of the disease, the better the outcome. The number one goal of treatment is to stop or slow progression of the disease, as over time, the inflammatory-adhesive process will entrap more and more nerve roots. This leads to bladder, gastrointestinal, sex organ, and lower extremity dysfunction and increased spinal fluid flow obstruction. Prevention of paraplegia is a paramount goal since the inflammatory-adhesive mass in the spinal canal may solidify, scar, and essentially sever neurologic connections to the lower extremities.[78] The second goal of treatment is to provide enough pain relief so the afflicted person can physically and mentally function, participate in activities of daily living, and have a reasonable quality of life. Some permanent recovery of neurologic function and reduction of pain is a third goal. Accomplishment of this goal is being observed more and more, particularly when the disease is caught and treated in its early stages. Almost total recovery has been observed in some cases.

TABLE: GOALS OF TREATMENT

1. Slow/stop progression of disease
2. Pain relief for comfort and function
3. Recovery to reduce neurologic impairments

Note: The best success in achieving goals is early diagnosis and treatment of AA.

21. CHRONIC CARE REQUIRED

AA now joins diseases such as diabetes, emphysema, and heart failure as chronic illnesses that require on-going care. Many measures used to treat other chronic diseases are applicable to AA. For example, the family should be involved in treatment, and the patient may benefit from self-help groups and psychologic support. Regular visits to the patient's medical practitioners are vital. In the case of AA, the patient and family may have to learn how to use some injectable medications for inflammation control and pain relief. This is particularly applicable to the use of treatment agents such as ketorolac (Toradol®), methylprednisolone, dexamethasone, and opioids.

There are some pharmacologic agents that have been reported to reduce or suppress neuroinflammation and warrant clinical trials.[61,64,66,98] They include minocycline, acetazolamide, pentoxifylline, and metformin. Some hormones are now known to be produced in the central nervous system and are called neurosteroids. They are described in more detail in a later chapter. At the time this handbook is written, we have begun to use them in treatment of AA, and now believe they are essential in long term care. Another emerging development in chronic care of the AA patient is autoimmune-suppression and antiviral therapy. For example, we are aware that some AA cases are now being treated with a variety of autoimmune-anti-inflammatory agents and antivirals such as acyclovir. At the time of this writing, however, we regret that our specific recommendations only cover initial and emergency care. Long-term care management of the AA patient needs considerable investigation, study, and evaluation.

22. THE BLOOD BRAIN BARRIER DICTATES TREATMENT

For a pharmacologic agent to be effective in treating AA, it must cross the blood brain barrier and enter the spinal fluid. This is apparently the reason that some pharmacologic agents used in RA and other non-spinal canal, inflammatory diseases are not effective in AA. For example, AA patients don't respond well to the anti-inflammation agents, ibuprofen, and naproxen. The anti-inflammatories, ketorolac (Toradol®) and diclofenac, however, are usually effective in AA apparently because they cross the blood brain barrier and enter the spinal fluid in significant enough concentrations to be effective. Only the corticosteroid, methylprednisolone and dexamethasone, as opposed to prednisone, hydrocortisone, and triamcinolone have proven to be very effective in treating AA, as they cross the blood brain barrier.

Interestingly, some non-prescription herbal anti-inflammatories, hormones, and nutritional agents are reported by AA patients to be effective. Their ability to cross the blood brain barrier is a likely reason why some natural agents are sometimes superior to some commercially made, synthetic agents.

23. THREE KEY ELEMENTS OF AA TREATMENT

Without treatment, AA is a most serious, debilitating, and life-shortening disease. We recommend that AA treatment consist of these three elements: (1) nutritional, (2) physiologic, and (3) pharmacologic. A key point emphasized here is that AA is still thought of and treated as if it is strictly a "pain problem." While pain relief is a necessary element of care, symptomatic pain treatment does not control inflammation, promote neurogenesis, or prevent progression of AA.

TABLE: THREE KEY ELEMENTS OF AA TREATMENT WITH EXAMPLES

NUTRITION	PHYSIOLOGIC	PHARMACOLOGIC
A. Vitamins B-12, C, D-3	A. Spinal fluid flow exercises Example: rocking	A. Spinal canal inflammation control Examples: ketorolac, methylprednisolone
B. High protein, Anti-inflammation diet	B. Neurologic maintenance Examples: stretching and walking	B. Regeneration of damaged tissues Examples: DHEA, nandrolone
C. Protein or collagen supplements	C. Electricity control Example: water soaking	C. Pain control Examples: low dose naltrexone, palmitoylethanolamide (PEA)

Note: The three elements of AA treatment require family support and self-care by the patient. Patients and family must become educated on the role of each element. Additional details of each element are described in subsequent chapters.

24. STARTING MEDICAL PROTOCOL

We recommend a three-component medical protocol to treat AA. Here are our starting recommendations which can and will undoubtably need to be revised as a patient is followed, over time.

Component One – Suppression of Spinal Canal Inflammation and Autoimmunity

a. Diclofenac 50 mg, 2 to 3 times daily
b. Ketorolac 10-30 mg by injection, oral, or nasal administration on a weekly or bimonthly basis
c. Methylprednisolone (Options)
    1. Oral-2 to 4 mg on 2 to 3 days a week
    2. Injection weekly or bimonthly, 10-20 mg

Component Two –Regeneration of Tissue

a. Dehydroepiandrosterone (DHEA) 25 to 75 mg daily
b. Nutritional measures- daily
    1. High protein, anti-inflammatory diet
    2. Protein-collagen supplement
    3. Vitamin C, 2000 to 4000 mg
    4. Vitamins: B_{12}, D_3
    5. Minerals: choice of one or more: magnesium, selenium, boron

c. Physiologic measures- daily
   1. Walks with arm swings
   2. Water soaks
   3. Stretching and extending legs, feet, and arms
   4. Rocking

Component Three – Pain Control

a. Low dose naltrexone* (LDN) 0.5 to 1.0 mg given twice a day
b. Neuropathic agent, choice: diazepam, clonazepam, gabapentin, carisoprodol, pregabalin
c. Bed-time sedative if needed: amitriptyline 25 to 50 mg
d. Palmitoylethanolamide (PEA) for pain flares

*Special notes:

1. LDN cannot be started in a person who takes daily opioids. Continue opioids if this is the case. Maximal LDN dose is 7.0mg twice a day.
2. Oral ketorolac must be taken with food or antacid. Daily use not recommended.
3. Shown here is the starting protocol. Follow-up will undoubtedly require changes in dosage and/or treatment agents, and the addition of other measures.

25. EMERGENCY TREATMENT AFTER SPINAL TAP OR EPIDURAL INJECTION

In unusual cases, symptoms suggesting AA may occur after a spinal tap or epidural injection (therapeutic or obstetrical). These symptoms may be the early development of AA. They may include lumbar pain, headaches, burning sensations, dizziness, leg weakness, and bladder dysfunction. Spinal fluid leaks or blood in the spinal canal are often suspected in these cases. Regardless, if symptoms indicate the possibility that AA may be developing, we recommend emergency treatment to hopefully prevent the development of AA.

A problem that we have routinely discovered is that medical practitioners commonly have the false belief that they can see AA on an MRI when symptoms begin or within a few hours or days after a spinal tap or epidural injection. Following a spinal tap or epidural injection, AA does not show on an MRI for at least four to six weeks. Consequently, emergency treatment must be started on history and symptoms rather than on MRI findings.

At the "First International Congress on Arachnoiditis and Tarlov Cysts (2010)," the physicians, Donna Holder and Antonio Aldrete, recommended that methylprednisolone 500 mg be given intravenously every day for five days as an emergency treatment. Since then, we are aware that a variety of intravenous methylprednisolone infusions with different dosages and frequency have been used by physicians as emergency treatment to prevent AA. Dr. Aldrete opined that intravenous methylprednisolone is only effective in preventing AA if given within about 60 days after the spinal tap or epidural.

We have used the following alternative protocol to intravenous methylprednisolone:

1. Medrol® (methylprednisolone) six-day oral dose pack
2. Ketorolac 30 to 60 mg injection for three consecutive days
3. Medroxyprogesterone 10 mg given twice a day for six days

In some, but not all cases, symptoms will abate during the week that either intravenous methylprednisolone or the alternative protocol shown above are administered. In most cases, however, symptoms reduce but don't totally abate. The reason for this is unclear, but a reasonable assumption is that spinal canal inflammation cannot be totally reversed once symptoms begin.

If pain and other symptoms don't totally abate, we recommend that the patient begin the three-component medical protocol described in the previous chapter. Patients with AA should remain in medical treatment until and if their pain and other symptoms resolve.

It is unclear why only a small percentage of persons who have spinal taps or epidural injections develop AA. It is also unknown why symptoms that begin after these procedures usually don't abate.

26. FOLLOW-UP AND FAMILY SUPPORT

AA must be looked at as a chronic disease that requires on-going care as does diabetes, schizophrenia, and asthma. Listed here are some of the author's tips, ideas, and experiences that may help in the chronic care of these patients.

- Frequent visits: Once treatment is initiated the patient will need to attend the practitioner's office at frequent intervals.

- Family involvement: The family can help in not only calming the fears that patients have with this disease, but they can also discipline and encourage the patient to engage in the nutritional and physiologic measures that are necessary to prevent progression of the disease and its deterioration. Too often the patient will overly focus on pain relief and self-pity.

- Office injections: Patients who come to the medical practitioner's office for their ketorolac, corticosteroid, or hormone injections simply do better. First, compliance with critical medications can be monitored, and the patient gets the support and empathy of the medical team.

- Objective laboratory testing: Depending on the patient's financial and insurance capability, periodic blood tests for inflammatory-autoimmune markers, hormones, and glucose levels are advisable as they aid in making clinical decisions. ESR, CRP, and cytokine panels on a periodic basis are essential to monitor spinal canal inflammation.

- Social support: Patients with AA commonly join social media support groups. They tend to be supportive, and the leaders of the groups are usually well-informed about the disease.

- Psychologic support: There is a trend among some psychologists to specialize in chronic disease management. They can be very helpful in the long-term case management of persons with AA. Persons with AA, if detected before severe complications set in, can often function well enough to work and socialize if encouraged to do so. Some psychologists are very adept at making this happen. Psychologic therapy can help those in the severe and catastrophic stages of AA find some happiness and quality of life.

- Risk/benefits of medication: AA is arguably the most debilitating spine and pain condition of modern times. It is objectively documented by contrast MRI. Deterioration, disease progression, and premature death is the fate if adequate pharmacologic therapy is not provided. Fears about the complications and risks of corticosteroids, benzodiazepines, anti-inflammatories, anabolic steroids and opioids may be valid, but the tragic person with MRI-documented AA is clinically, ethically, and legally eligible for medications that may have risks. With informed consent, the benefits of drugs with risks almost always outweigh the risks in an AA patient.

- Neuroinflammatory Medications: These agents have been shown in laboratory testing to reduce neuroinflammation: pentoxifylline, acetazolamide, minocycline, metformin. A short clinical trial of any one of these agents may prove helpful.

- Ancillary Medical Service: At the time of this writing ancillary medical services and personnel including physical and massage therapists, chiropractors, and nurses likely know little about AA. Some therapists and chiropractors have actually injured patients with AA because they are not familiar with the pathologic consequences of spinal canal inflammation, nerve root entrapment, spinal fluid flow obstruction and spinal fluid leakage. In particular they are not aware that the diseased and weakened spinal canal covering can be over-stretched or torn. Medical personnel must be community educators until there is widespread knowledge about AA. In particular, it is hazardous to stretch the spine or put excess pressure on it. For example, weightlifting must be restricted to no more than about three to ten pounds. It appears that any excess strain on the spine can injure the spinal canal covering as it is inflamed, porous, and has a lack of tensile strength. With the caveats listed here, stretching, strengthening, massage, and other measures that enhance blood flow and build tissue can be beneficial.

27. NUTRITIONAL MEASURES FOR AA

Presented here are nutritional measures to help control pain, regenerate damaged tissues, and promote healing of AA. Collagen and the neurotransmitters that control pain are made from the protein that one eats. AA is a spinal canal inflammatory disease, so a daily intake of anti-inflammatory foods is essential. Also, high blood glucose (sugar) causes pain to increase. Here are our recommendations to patients.

1. Eat one or more of these protein foods each day: eggs, cottage cheese, beef, pork, fish/seafood, chicken, turkey.

2. Eat some of these anti-inflammatory fruits and vegetables each day.
    - ✓ Fruits: berries (any kind), apple, peach, plum
    - ✓ Vegetables: broccoli, Brussel sprouts, avocado, beets, carrots, cucumber, celery, leaf greens, squash, tomatoes, zucchini

3. Limit sugar and starches:
    - ✓ Use sugar substitutes and sugar free drinks
    - ✓ Eliminate milk and fruit juices
    - ✓ Minimize these high-sugar, starch, or gluten foods: bread, pastries, potatoes, pies, cakes, pizza, corn, noodles, pasta, pancakes
    - ✓ Check blood sugar to see if it is in normal range

4. Daily nutrients:

- ✓ Vitamin C, 2000 to 4000 mg a day
- ✓ Minerals, use one or more: magnesium, selenium, boron
- ✓ B-12, D-3
- ✓ Collagen or protein supplement
- ✓ Vitamin-mineral tablet/capsule

TABLE: SUMMARY OF NUTRITIONAL MEASURES

- ✓ Daily protein
- ✓ Daily anti-inflammatory vegetables and fruits
- ✓ Limit high sugar, starch, gluten foods
- ✓ Drink only sugar free liquids
- ✓ Daily supplements
    - Protein/collagen
    - Vitamin C, 2000-4000 mg
    - Vitamin B-12, D-3
    - Choice: magnesium, selenium, boron
    - Vitamin/mineral preparation

Note: Patients with AA often have such severe pain that it is their only focus. Medical Practitioners and family members must encourage and educate on the necessity to participate in specific daily nutritional and physiologic measures in order to slow or prevent AA from progressing.

28. SPINAL FLUID FLOW EXERCISES

Exercises to promote and activate spinal fluid flow is a new concept in treatment of AA. Spinal fluid turns over (made anew) about every 4 to 6 hours.[23] Its normal functions include lubrication of nerve roots to prevent friction and inflammation, carry nutrients including medications to the cauda equina, and wash out biologic-metabolic waste and toxic materials such as inflammation particles.[57] AA is a mass in the spinal canal that disturbs both the rate and volume of spinal fluid flow. Consequently, patients may experience symptoms in their upper extremities and head.[102]

In the mid-1950's, former President John F. Kennedy (JFK) had severe pain, required crutches, and was desperate to the point of giving up his political career after failing to get relief with multiple back surgeries. Some say he even considered suicide. He was referred to Janet Travel, MD, one of the most noted pain and rehabilitation specialists of the day. She hospitalized JFK and brought a rocking chair into his room and prescribed rocking several times a day. JFK continued regular rocking right into the White House. Several photographs taken during this time popularized rocking chair therapy. Since the days of JFK, not much has been said or written about the health benefits of rocking. This is likely because there has not been, until now, a plausible, possible explanation as to why rocking has a health benefit. Rocking may enhance or speed up spinal fluid flow around an AA mass, as well as enhance lymphatic flow.

Walking or slight bouncing on a trampoline may enhance spinal fluid flow. For example, patients will often experience nasal dripping when they begin to walk on a trampoline.

Although there is no statistical evidence that spinal fluid flow exercises benefit AA patients, clinical experience compels us to recommend the following exercises to enhance spinal fluid flow:

TABLE: SPINAL FLUID FLOW EXERCISES

- Walking or slight bouncing on a trampoline
- Daily walking with arm swings
- Rocking chair or swinging on a porch swing
- Deep breathing

Note: Spinal fluid provides nutrients for healing and flushes out inflammatory particles and other biologic wastes. We highly recommend the above exercise, as we believe they benefit the AA patient.

PICTURE: PRESIDENT JOHN F. KENNEDY IN ROCKING CHAIR WITH SEAT CUSHION

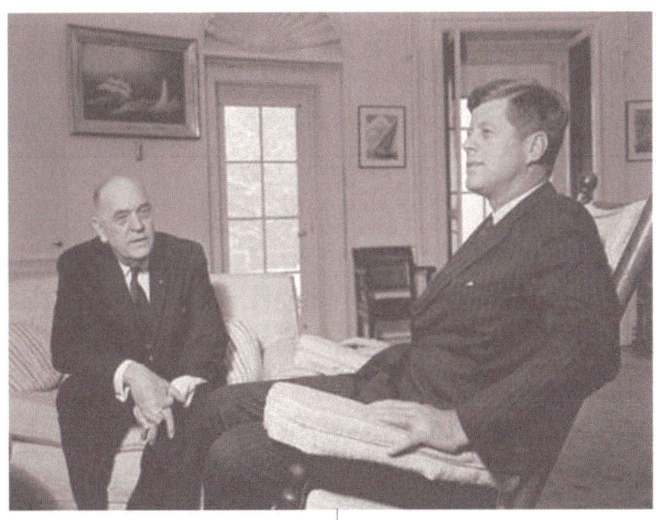

Note: President John F. Kennedy, meeting Dr. William Menninger, in his famous rocking chair and seat cushion in the Oval Office. All patients with AA are advised to follow the lead of JFK.

29. EYE, EAR, NASAL SYMPTOMS WITH AA

Eye, hearing, and nasal symptoms with AA are common. They include blurred vision (spots), ear ringing (tinnitus), funny smells, nasal watering, and headaches or pressure sensations in the head. We believe that the major cause of eye, ear, and nasal symptoms is spinal fluid flow obstruction or impairment since AA acts as a mass in the lower spinal canal and also causes stasis of fluid in the lower spinal canal which interferes with normal flow.[102] Many persons afflicted with AA and their medical practitioners may believe that a patients eye, ear, and nasal symptoms are only caused by spinal fluid leaks, because they are not aware that symptoms may also be caused by spinal fluid flow impairment. Both spinal fluid flow obstruction and spinal fluid leakage occur with AA. We recommend that every person with eye, ear, and nasal symptoms have a 5-day trial of acetazolamide. Start with 125 mg orally for 2 consecutive days and then go to 250 mg a day. If acetazolamide helps, it can be taken "as needed" or on a regular on-going basis up to 500 mg a day.

Acetazolamide, in addition to lowering spinal fluid pressure, suppresses neuroinflammation. Consequently, some AA patients find it to be very therapeutic in that it reduces pain and other neurologic symptoms such as bladder dysfunction and burning sensations.

30. PAIN FLARE TREATMENT

Most pain flares are apparently caused by a surge in inflammation inside the spinal canal. Flares are often due to overexertion or overextension of the spinal canal due to excess walking, weightlifting, or sitting, but many occur for no known reason. Flares should be interpreted to mean that inflammation has erupted which may cause more damage to cauda equina nerve roots and the arachnoid-dural covering of the spinal canal. Consequently, flares should be considered emergencies to be curtailed as soon as possible to prevent additional tissue damage and disease progression.

AA flares are usually best treated with injectable ketorolac (Toradol®) 30 to 60 mg, and/or injectable methylprednisolone (Medrol®) 10 to 20 mg, or dexamethasone 5 to 10 mg. Extra pain relief can be obtained with an injection of hydromorphone (4 to 10 mg), meperidine (50 to 100 mg), or morphine (10 to 20 mg). Opioid suppositories are excellent. Injections of ketorolac and methylprednisolone can be safely administered for two consecutive days. A 6-day Medrol® (methylprednisolone) Oral Dose Pak may be adequate for mild to moderate flares.

Water soaking with Epsom Salts, ice packs, magnet rubs, and electromagnetic energy administration may also assist emergency flare treatment.

31. PALLIATIVE CARE FOR LATE-STAGE AA

Unfortunately, there are long-term patients with AA who have never been diagnosed or treated for the disease. Consequently, their disease has progressed to the severe or catastrophic stage. They are extremely debilitated, and some are bed-bound. They have never had the benefits of inflammation control or tissue regeneration therapies. Most have had multiple surgeries, epidural injections, and other therapies in the past but to little avail. Many of these individuals have MRIs that show dense scarring of nerve root clumps, and even calcification.[85] The lower spinal canal may be distended ("empty sac appearance") and/or show spinal fluid flow obstruction. Such complications as urinary and bowel incontinence, paralysis, and dementia may be present. Urine catheterization and diapers may be necessary. In these tragic individuals, palliative care to provide intractable pain relief and end-of-life comfort is essential. Anti-inflammatory, tissue regeneration, and nutritional and physiologic measures may be ineffective as cauda equina nerve roots may be irrevocably damaged. Measures including high dose or injectable opioids, implanted electrical stimulators, or intrathecal opioid administration may be warranted in these cases. Families need to be told if the palliative stage is present, so they don't have false hopes about recovery with the AA treatment that is effective in the mild to moderate cases.

Pain in these cases may be constant and incapacitating. Our recommendation for opioid therapy is injectable hydromorphone or fentanyl by the patch or nasal routes. A dopaminergic agent such as amphetamine salts (Adderall®) or methylphenidate (Ritalin®) and a neuropathic agent such as gabapentin, pregabalin, or clonazepam may be necessary to obtain pain control. Adrenal support with a corticoid may be necessary.

AA patients who are in the mild to moderate stages or categories of this disease need, along with their family, to be educated that this disease can progress into the severe or catastrophic categories. A major goal of early diagnosis and treatment of patients in the mild or moderate stages of AA is to prevent or at least slow progression to the severe and catastrophic stages.

32. KETOROLAC (TORADOL®) ESSENTIAL FOR MOST PERSONS WITH AA

Ketorolac (Toradol®) is almost an "essential" treatment agent in AA. Diclofenac and indomethacin have been the only other anti-inflammatory agents to be effective, but only in some cases. The majority of persons with AA report ketorolac to relieve pain and reduce other symptoms. For incompletely known reasons it is the most effective anti-inflammatory drug other than corticosteroids for AA. Apparently this agent crosses the blood brain barrier, enters spinal fluid, and attaches to critical receptors in the spinal cord and brain better than other currently available anti-inflammatory drugs. A reason why a single injection of ketorolac may provide pain relief for several days is that it suppresses the n-methyl-D-aspartate (NMDA) receptor in the central nervous system.

We recommend that ketorolac be started on a weekly or bimonthly basis at a dose of 10 to 30 mg. Oral 10 mg tablets are available, and a single tablet usually doesn't cause gastrointestinal bleeding if taken with food or antacids. Ketorolac injections, if well-tolerated, can be given in 30 to 60 mg dosages. Due to the risk of gastrointestinal bleeding and renal toxicity, ketorolac (Toradol®) must be used with specific precautions. It cannot be taken for five consecutive days. As long as days are not consecutive, it can be taken intermittently over a long period. We do not normally recommend it be used more than two consecutive days unless for severe pain flares. Patients need to be educated to look for black stools or bloody vomitus if they use ketorolac. A hemoglobin, creatinine, and blood urea nitrogen (BUN) are recommended about every six months.

Patients and families can be taught to give at-home injections of ketorolac, or they can be given in the practitioner's office. Ketorolac can usually be simultaneously administered with cyanocobalamin (B_{12}). A corticosteroid or opioid can be used on the same day for severe pain flares. Normally, however, we recommend that corticosteroids be used on days that ketorolac is not used.

If used by persons over 70 years of age, there must be regular monitoring for gastrointestinal bleeding. A nasal formulation is now available, and it appears to be a safe substitute or even preferable formulation over the injectable or oral forms.

33. SELECT CORTICOSTEROIDS FOR AA

AA is a most serious spinal canal inflammatory disease. Its morbidity and mortality is such that medical practitioners are well justified in using pharmacologic agents, such as corticosteroids and ketorolac, that have well known risks and complications. Until and if specific biologic agents are identified for AA as with rheumatoid arthritis, select corticosteroids given on a low dose, intermittent basis are almost essential to control AA.[49,55,61,63,90]

Methylprednisolone and dexamethasone are the preferred corticosteroids because they cross the blood brain barrier, enter spinal fluid, and act on micro glial cells.[49,66,90,98] Prednisone, triamcinolone, and hydrocortisone have little or no effect on AA.

Since corticosteroids given on a regular basis cause the well-known complications of osteoporosis and Cushing's Syndrome, it is recommended they only be given on a low dose, intermittent basis, with days skipped between dosages. One of these two basic regimens is recommended as a starting point:

1. Oral dosage on 2 to 3 days a week

- Methylprednisolone, 2 to 4 mg
- Dexamethasone, 0.25 to 0.50 mg

2. Weekly or bimonthly injection

- Methylprednisolone, 10 to 20 mg
- Dexamethasone, 2.5 to 5.0 mg

Patients and family can be taught to give at-home corticosteroid injections, or the patient can attend the practitioner's office. Vitamin B_{12} and other medications can usually be mixed in the same syringe with either methylprednisolone or dexamethasone.

Methylprednisolone has been, in our hands, more consistently effective than dexamethasone. There are some patients, however, who respond better to dexamethasone than methylprednisolone. If an on-going patient is not responding well to treatment, a switch of these two corticosteroids is recommended. For unclear reasons some patients only respond to one but not the other.

34. LOW DOSE NALTREXONE: FIRST PAIN CONTROL DRUG OF CHOICE

Naltrexone in low doses (LDN) is the initial pain control drug of preference in persons with AA. The reason is that it simultaneously provides pain relief, suppression of inflammation and autoimmunity, and promotes neurogenesis. The starting dose is 0.5 to 1.0 mg given twice a day. If pain relief is not satisfactory, raise the dose intermittently over 4 to 6 weeks. The average dose is about 4.0 mg given twice a day. The maximum dose we have observed is 14 mg a day taken 7.0 mg in the morning and evening. Administration is usually daily, but it can be taken on only 3 to 5 days a week in mild cases of AA. It can be taken as a single daily dose if more effective than a split dosage. Ketorolac and/or one of the corticosteroids, methylprednisolone or dexamethasone, and all non-opioid pain relievers can be taken with it. The analgesic-nutritional drug, palmitoylethanolamide (PEA), is a normal body biochemical that is highly recommended for flares in patients who take LDN as it, like LDN, has analgesic, anti-inflammatory, and neurogenic properties.

Few side-effects or drug interactions have been observed with LDN, but a few patients have been unable to take it due to dysphoria, headache, vertigo, or nausea. Persons who are on daily opioids cannot be started on naltrexone as significant withdrawal symptoms may occur. Some persons who are on a stable dose of LDN can safely take for pain flares, an occasional low dose of opioids such as tramadol, codeine, hydromorphone, or hydrocodone.

Buprenorphine (Subutex®, Suboxone®) is an agonist-antagonist opioid formulation that has many of the benefits and attributes of LDN. It is a good choice if LDN doesn't adequately control pain as buprenorphine is usually a more potent reliever that is LDN. If LDN or buprenorphine don't adequately control pain, standard opioid therapy will be necessary.

35. NEUROSTEROIDS FOR TREATMENT OF AA

One of the great research discoveries of the past generation is that the central nervous system makes a specific set of hormones called neurosteroids.[19,32,58,77,84] Their function is to suppress neuroinflammation and regrow damaged nerve tissue.[8,37] Great clinical interest in the use of neurosteroids evolved when veterans who served in the military after September 11, 2001 were found to have significantly greater pain when neurosteroids dropped in their blood.[58] We have found, in our experience, that some neurosteroids appear to greatly benefit AA patients. We have chosen DHEA as the neurosteroid of choice in our starting protocol. DHEA has been shown to have neuroregenerative properties and has been shown in controlled studies to be effective in systemic lupus and rheumatoid arthritis.[8,15,30,50,79,84] DHEA has direct actions on inflammation and neurogenesis. It is also a precursor to estradiol, testosterone, and nandrolone. Progesterone has been shown to protect neuronal cells, extinguish neuroinflammation, and heal spinal cord damage.[20,27,40,101] We advocate a short course of medroxyprogesterone in our emergency protocol.

We realize that there is a paucity of controlled studies with neurosteroids, but feel with informed consent, that short trials in AA patients are warranted. The use of neurosteroids in animal studies can only be described as "amazing." For example, spinal cord severance in rats has been treated with pregnenolone and human chorionic gonadotropin (HCG).[36] Almost total reversal has occurred. Neuroinflammation and apoptosis has been reversed with progesterone, DHEA, testosterone, and estrogen.[20,40] Use of neurosteroids in humans for suppression of neuroinflammation and regeneration of damaged tissue is limited at this time. Positive results have, however, been reported with progesterone treatment of stroke and traumatic brain injury, DHEA in treatment of systemic lupus, and estrogen in rheumatoid arthritis.[15,17,21,27,30,33,79,101]

Our use of neurosteroids has been quite effective in patients who have stabilized on the three-component medical protocol presented in a previous chapter. Human chorionic gonadotropin (HCG) has been, in our hands, a beneficial anabolic hormone.[91, 92] HCG consists of two biologic units.[60] One raises blood levels of progesterone, estrogen, and testosterone. The other unit is a specific neural tissue anabolic agent.[72,73] We have observed reduction of pain, decreased use of opioid drugs, less urinary dysfunction, and improved strength of lower extremities with HCG. Absent controlled clinical data, we recommend a short trial of HCG for one month. Starting dosage is 250 to 500 units 2 to 3 times a week taken by injection or buccal routes.

Besides HCG, we have found medroxyprogesterone, DHEA, estradiol, pregnenolone, and testosterone to be beneficial in selected patients. When these hormones are used, we recommend a one-month trial. If no effect or side effects occur, stop the neurosteroid.

Nandrolone is a testosterone derivative classified as an anabolic steroid and labeled for wasting, debilitating diseases. It is a naturally produced neurosteroid and found in serum at low concentrations. It is likely derived from DHEA or testosterone. Early trials with a dose of 25 to 50 mg once or twice a day on three to five days a week are being used as this handbook is written. Early results appear promising in that pain appears reduced, multiple neurologic functions have improved, and deterioration of AA has appeared to arrest or be greatly retarded.

Interestingly, two non-prescription, over-the-counter, hormonal agents have become popular with AA patients. One is colostrum and the other is a deer antler substance called "velvet." Some species of deer grow a pituitary-like substance in their antlers that can be harvested and safely formulated for human use. These two agents consist of multiple neurosteroids.

In summary, neurosteroids are a new concept. Some appear promising in the prevention and treatment of AA. Given the severity and catastrophic ramifications of AA, short clinical trials with informed consent appear warranted.

36. NEUROPATHIC PAIN IN AA

"Neuropathic" is a term that has recently been adopted in pain treatment circles to classify a specific type of pain and a class of drugs that control it.[66,98] The term "neuropathic" simply means nerve-damage or impairment. With nerve damage or impairment, the normal flow of electricity is interrupted. When electricity cannot normally flow, it accumulates in one spot and will cause pain and inflammation. AA is a nerve root entrapment disease that causes "neuropathic" pain. Consequently, the following complications among others may occur: paralysis of lower extremities, urinary, gastrointestinal, and sexual dysfunction, jerking or stabbing pains, sensations of water dripping or insects crawling, and burning feet.

The natural chemical in nerves that conducts the flow of electricity is called "gamma amino butyric acid" (hereafter GABA). Drugs classified as "neuropathic" are synthetic derivatives or analogues of GABA. They either substitute for GABA or enhance its natural functions. Some of the most popular neuropathic drugs are gabapentin, carisoprodol (Soma®), baclofen, diazepam (Valium®), pregabalin (Lyrica®), and topiramate (Topamax®). Natural non-prescription neuropathic agents include valerian root, glutamine, ashwagandha, and pure GABA (taken under the tongue).

One or more neuropathic drugs are usually essential in AA to keep electricity flowing and control pain.[66] Natural neuropathic agents can be combined with prescription agents, to possibly provide better relief.

37. LOW DOSE, INTERMITTENT ADMINISTRATION OF MOST CONSISTENT AGENTS

AA is a terrible debilitating disease that causes great suffering and shortened lifespan if not aggressively treated. Unfortunately, few pharmacologic agents have shown effectiveness in AA, and those that have been the most consistent may have side effects if used on a high dose, regular basis. In our hands four agents have shown consistent positive treatment results. It is recommended that these four not be shunned but used on a low dose, intermittent basis to achieve effectiveness while avoiding side effects.

Agent 1 – Ketorolac (Toradol®): This agent cannot be given for over five consecutive days due to renal toxicity and gastrointestinal bleeding. We recommend a 10 to 60 mg dose by injection, oral, or nasal route to be initially given once weekly, or to be even more cautious, once every two weeks. A more frequent dosage schedule can be used if the patient tolerates it.

Agent 2 – Corticosteroid: The most consistent corticosteroid has been methylprednisolone. For safety, it can usually be given one to three times a week at an oral dose of 2 to 4 mg. Dexamethasone is the best alternative to methylprednisolone, and some AA patients respond better to it. The same dosage frequency applies to dexamethasone at an oral dose of 0.5 to 0.75 mg.

Another low dose, intermittent strategy is a monthly or bimonthly injection of methylprednisolone or dexamethasone. The recommended dosage of methylprednisolone is 10 to 20 mg and that of dexamethasone is 5 to 10 mg. Patients can be taught to give their own injections, or they can be given in the practitioner's office.

Agent 3 – Human Chorionic Gonadotropin (HCG): This hormone is a potent neurogenic, anabolic agent.[60,72,73,91] It elevates estrogen, testosterone, and progesterone and it, by itself, produces neurogenesis. In our hands, this agent has been associated with recovery from partial leg paralysis or lowering back pain to a point that opioids were not required.[92] Starting dose is 250 to 500 units on 2 to 3 days a week. The dosage can be raised over time if necessary. We recommend a one-month trial, to determine if it is safe and effective.

Agent 4 – Low Dose Naltrexone (LDN): This agent provides pain relief, suppresses inflammation and autoimmunity, and promotes neurogenesis. Starting dose is 0.5 to 1.0 mg given twice a day. The maximum dose we have observed is 7.0 mg twice a day. LDN is usually taken daily but can be used on a less frequent schedule such as 3 to 5 days a week. An occasional low dose opioid such as tramadol, codeine, or hydrocodone can usually be taken with LDN to control pain flares.

Special Note: Although other pharmacologic agents are known by us to have therapeutic value in selected patients, the four agents listed here, when taken on a low dose, intermittent basis, have provided the most consistent benefits and superior outcomes.

38. THERAPEUTIC TEST FOR INFLAMMATION

Unfortunately, blood levels of inflammatory markers do not always reflect the presence of inflammation in the spinal canal. A good test to determine if active inflammation is present is an injection of ketorolac (30 to 60 mg) or methylprednisolone (10 to 20 mg). A 6-Day Medrol® Dose Pak (methylprednisolone) that reduces pain and inflammation is also a therapeutic test. If the patient experiences some pain relief, it means that inflammation is present and requires on-going medical suppression. If the patient improves, a therapeutic, on-going anti-inflammatory treatment program with ketorolac or methylprednisolone is recommended. If the patient doesn't respond to the test agents, one can reasonably assume that pain is primarily due to irreversible nerve root damage and dysfunction ("Neuropathy") rather than active inflammation. Also, a lack of positive response to the test agent may mean that inflammation is simply in remission and may later return.

Given the serious tissue-destructive properties of spinal canal inflammation, it is prudent to continuously attempt to suppress it. For example, there are a number of herbal or natural agents including curcumin, serrapeptase, astragalus, and whole adrenal gland that are quite safe and popular with AA patients. Medical practitioners may wish to recommend one or more of these agents as a precautionary measure to suppress inflammation.

39. EXPERIMENTAL AND INVESTIGATIONAL THERAPIES

A fair number of researchers and investigators are attempting new treatments for AA. Among the prominent efforts are stem cell administration, intravenous infusions of various nutritional, hormonal, and enzymatic agents, and a surgical procedure called thecaloscopy. The latter is an attempt to dislodge or free up adhesions and improve spinal fluid flow. A number of pharmacologic agents that are already available on the commercial market are being given trials. These include hormonal and antiviral agents. A variety of electromagnetic and electro-current therapies are being studied. Medical practitioners should inform patients who wish to attempt invasive, investigational treatments including intravenous injections that there may be unknown risks. We approve of investigation and experimental procedures once a patient is stabilized on a three-component medical protocol that includes suppression of spinal canal inflammation, neurogenesis, and pain control. Why? If the investigational treatment doesn't work, what is the patient to do for on-going treatment? Maybe it partially works but other treatment is still needed. It is therefore prudent to have an ongoing, chronic care plan in place before attempting a "silver bullet" approach. Persons with AA must also be warned about over-promise and even fraudulent schemes to treat AA.

40. PHYSIOLOGIC MEASURES

AA is an inflammatory, nerve entrapment disease. Consequently, there are a few physiologic measures deemed essential to prevent progression and deterioration of AA. The first is that the patient must take intentional daily walks and do flexion and extension exercises of the arms, legs, and feet. Although it is somewhat unclear how these exercises prevent leg paralysis and foot drop, we believe they are preventive. Hopefully they also promote some relief and recovery. Next to daily walks and extremity flexion/extension exercises, we deem daily water soaking to be essential. Although tub, pool, and jacuzzi soaking may be optimal, warm showers will help. Water soaking, including foot baths, is therapy "of the ages" and its mechanism is debatable. We believe it eliminates retained or sequestered electricity that causes dysfunctional nerve conduction. This is also the apparent mechanism of magnets and the "centuries old" practice of wearing copper jewelry. Magnet rubs over the spine may also enhance spinal fluid flow. As with many physiologic measures, they are controversial and debatable, but many AA patients find these measures to be of benefit.

AA patients must sit on cushions as sitting may compress the spinal canal at the lumbar-sacral vertebral junction which is the usual location of an AA mass. Patients must be counseled to avoid sitting very long in a car or plane ride as they can over compress an AA mass and produce further neurologic damage. A soft back brace is recommended for extended walks such as shopping in a grocery store or retail center. There is also a risk of stumbling or falls that a brace may prevent.

Massage and heat applied to the lower back are old remedies that may increase blood flow and enhance spinal fluid flow. Electromagnetic and some electric current therapies may be very helpful, particularly in patients who have spinal fluid "seepage" or "leakage." Electromagnetic pulsed energy and micro electric currents may possibly penetrate two to four inches below the skin and reach the dural-arachnoid canal cover. If so, some permanent healing may occur.

Weightlifting must be restricted. A weight of no more than three to ten pounds is recommended. Why? The arachnoid-dural covering of the spinal canal is diseased and it cannot be overstretched or overstrained for fear of a tear at an AA site.

TABLE: PHYSIOLOGIC MEASURES FOR AA

- ✓ Seat cushions
- ✓ Soft back brace for extended walks
- ✓ Limit time sitting in one position
- ✓ Daily walks
- ✓ Daily arm, leg, and foot flexion and extension exercises
- ✓ Daily water soaking
- ✓ Magnet rubs and/or contact
- ✓ Copper jewelry
- ✓ Electro current therapy
- ✓ Electromagnetic energy therapy
- ✓ Massage
- ✓ Heat
- ✓ Light weightlifting (3 to 10 pounds)
- ✓ Rocking
- ✓ Trampoline walking

Note: The best physiologic measures are those that the patient will faithfully do every day.

41. TREATMENT OF SPINAL FLUID LEAKS

Small temporary leaks in the spinal canal covering seem to heal with the anti-inflammatory treatment recommended in the starting protocol. Larger leaks or chronic seepage may not only require anti-inflammatory agents, but corticosteroids and tissue regeneration measures. Electromagnetic energy and electric current therapies including lasers, pulsed radiofrequency energy, infrared, and transcutaneous electrical stimulation may not only relieve pain but assist with sealing a leak. They may also help heal tissues that are irritated by spinal fluid that has leaked out of the canal. Local treatment for soft tissue pain including anesthetic gels or patches may provide relief. In recalcitrant cases we recommend trials of one of these potent anabolic hormones: (1) testosterone, (2) human chorionic gonadotropin, or (3) nandrolone.

We do not recommend blood, or any other chemical agent be injected into the spinal canal of a patient with active AA. Our experience has been that blood or other substances aggravate the existing inflammatory-adhesive process that causes the arachnoid-dural covering to become overly porous and allow fluid to leak into the epidural space and paraspinal soft tissues.

SUMMARY

AA is a spinal canal inflammatory disease that occurs when cauda equina nerve roots become attached by adhesions to the inner wall of the arachnoid-dural (meninges) covering of the spinal canal. A clump or mass is formed in the inflammatory adhesive process that entraps nerve roots which primarily innervate the bladder, gastrointestinal tract, sex organs, and lower extremities. Parathesias of burning, water dripping, or insects crawling are common. Severe, intractable, and disabling pain may occur. The inflamed spinal canal covering may become porous and leak spinal fluid into paraspinal tissues. The mass inside the spinal canal usually interferes with spinal fluid flow and creates symptoms such as blurred vision, tinnitus, and headache. If untreated, AA is a progressive disease that may result in total incapacitation, malnutrition, dementia, paralysis, a bed bound state, adrenal failure, and early death.

In these modern times AA is almost always the end result of multiple, pathologic factors. The major factors today are structural spine abnormalities, genetic connective tissue diseases, autoimmune collagen disorders, trauma, and medical procedures.

Post viral autoimmune-collogen disorder due to the Epstein Barr virus (EBV) is apparently emerging as a major contributing factor.

AA is staged or categorized as mild, moderate, severe, or catastrophic. It is diagnosed by a typical set of symptoms or laboratory abnormalities, physical findings, and confirmed by a contrast MRI.

In the past AA has been considered a rare, hopeless disease that could not be treated. That belief no longer holds true. Treatment to date indicates that the disease, while incurable, is controllable, and some relief, recovery, and cessation or slowing of disease progression can be obtained for most patients.

AA is now being recognized in every community and medical practice that encounters patients with back pain. This handbook provides a "first generation" attempt to diagnose and treat this emerging disease. The future will inevitably bring about more understanding and improvements over the recommendations in this handbook.

GLOSSARY OF TERMS

Adhesive arachnoiditis: A spinal canal inflammatory disease in which there is a clump or mass of cauda equina nerve roots that are glued by adhesions to the arachnoid-dural covering of the spinal canal.

Adhesive arachnoiditis ossification: This term has been applied to cases that show calcification in the clump or mass of AA.[18]

Arachnoiditis-non-adhesive: Inflammation of the arachnoid membrane or layer of the spinal canal covering (meninges) without any nerve roots adhered or "glued" to it. This condition cannot specifically be identified by MRI. It is a clinical diagnosis based on signs, symptoms, and laboratory tests.

Axial view: "Toe-to-Head" view or images of the cauda equina and spinal canal. It is a cross section or pictorial "slice" of the spinal canal.

Canal distortion: The normal circular contour of the spinal canal has lost its normal shape due to some pathologic process such as fibrosis, scarring, or loss of tensile strength.

Cauda equina: About two dozen nerve roots that emanate from the spinal cord at about the level of thoracic 12(T-12) or lumbar 1 (L-1) and are suspended in spinal fluid.

Circular contour: Cauda equina nerve roots appear circular on the axial view of an MRI. Loss of circular contour represents edema, inflammation, or degeneration.

Clumping or coalescence: Multiple nerve roots have joined together due to inflammation and adhesion formation.

Contrast: The ability on an MRI to distinguish spinal fluid by white coloring from solid tissue which shows as varying shades of gray. This may be accomplished with intravenous dye or with high resolution imaging.

Disorganization: Severe displacement with gross distortion of the normal nerve root pattern.

Displacement: One or more nerve roots are moved or relocated to an abnormal position on axial (toe-to-head) MRI images.

Empty sac: The lower lumbar and/or sacral spinal canal is dilated with no sign of nerve roots passing through the interior of the canal. The cause is nerve roots being completely adhered and attached to the inside of the spinal canal covering rather than be free floating in the spinal fluid.

Lumbar levels: There are normally five lumbar vertebrae levels being designated L1 through L5 with L1 being the topmost vertebrae.

Meninges: This is the spinal canal covering in the lumbar-sacral region that primarily consists of an inside layer called arachnoid and an outer layer called the dura. The word "covering" is preferentially used in this handbook rather than meninges or theca to simplify understanding.

Peripheralization: Cauda equina nerve roots are adhered by adhesions to the inside of the spinal canal cover. This finding is often called "empty sac" as the canal may look empty on both axial and lateral views.

Sacral levels: Two sacral levels will be noted in this handbook. These vertebrae will be designated S1 and S2.

Sagittal View: This is the side or lateral MRI view of the spine.

Seepage: Spinal fluid that has leaked or seeped into tissues outside the spinal canal. Contrast MRI imaging shows spinal fluid as white.

Skin channels: Spinal fluid that has seeped through the arachnoid-dural cover of the spinal canal may work its way to the skin surface and form tracks or channels on the skin surface.

Spacing: This refers to the normal space between cauda equina nerve roots as seen on axial MRI images. The space appears as white between gray or black nerve roots. Spacing disappears with nerve root enlargement or coalescence.

Spinal canal: Also known as the thecal sac. The spinal canal is a structure like a closed pipe that carries the spinal fluid. The fluid is primarily produced in the brain and flows down the canal on one side and flows back up to the brain to be diverted into lymph nodes and the general blood and lymphatic systems. The word canal is preferentially used here to simplify understanding.

Symmetry and asymmetry: Cauda equina nerves are normally situated in a symmetrical position with half on the right and half on left sides of the spinal canal. Asymmetry means that some nerve roots have been displaced or shifted from their normal position due to a disease process.

Thickening: Cauda equina nerve roots have a rather standard thickness. Thickening or enlargement means the roots have edema, inflammation, and/or scarring.

REFERENCES

1. Addison T. 1855. *The constitutional and local effects of disease of the supra-renal capsules.* London: Samuel Highley.

2. Aldrete JA. 2003. *Arachnoiditis: the silent epidemic.* Mexico: Future Med Publishers,.

3. Aldrete JA. 2010. "History and evaluation of arachnoiditis:The evidence revealed." *Insurgentes Centro 51-A Col San Rafael* (Insurgentes Centro 51-A) p3-14.

4. Aldrete JA. 2006. "Suspecting and diagnosing arachnoiditis." *Pract Pain Mgt* 16:74-87.

5. Anderson TL, Morris JM, Wald JT, et al. 2017. "Imaging appearance of advanced chronic adhesive arachnoiditis: A retrospective review." *Am J Roentgenol* 209:648-655.

6. Andersson GB. 1999. "Epidemiological features of chronic low back pain." *Lancet* 354:582-585.

7. Baber J, Erdek M,. 2016. "Failed back surgery syndrome: current perspectives." *J Pain Res* 9:979-987.

8. Baulieu EE, Robel P,. 1998. "Dehydroepiandrosterone (DHEA) and dehydroepiandrosterone sulfate (DHEAS) as neuroactive neurosteroids." *Proc Natl Acad Sci* 95:4089-4091.

9. Bilello J, Tennant F,. 2016. "Patterns of chronic inflammation in extensively treated patients with arachnoiditis and chronic intractable pain." *Postgrad Med* 92:1-5.

10. Bjornevik, et al.s. 2022. "Longitudinal analysis reveals high prevalence of Epstein-Barr virus associated with multiple sclerosi." *Science* DoI:10.1126/science.abj8222.

11. Bourne IH. 1990. "Lumbo-sacral adhesive arachnoiditis: A review." *J R Soc Med* 83:262-265.

12. Burton C. 1978. " Lumbosacral arachnoiditis." *Spine* 3:24-30.

13. Castori M, Voorman NC. 2014. "Neurologic manifestations of Ehlers-Danlos Syndrome(s): a review." *Iran J Neuro* 13:190-208.

14. Chang CW, Peng P,. 2011. "Failed back surgery syndrome." *Pain Med* 12:577-606.

15. Chang DM, Chu SJ, Chen HC, et al. 2004. "Dehydroepiandrosterone suppresses interleukin 10 synthesis in women with systemic lupus erythematosus." *Ann Rheum Dis* 63:1623-1620.

16. Charcot JM, Joffrey A,. 1869. "Deax cas d'atrophic musculaire progressive avec lesions de a substance gris et des faisceaux anterolateraux de la moelle spinaire." *Arch de Physiologic* 2:354-358.

17. Cirillo DJ, Wallace RB, Wu L, et al. 2006. "Effects of hormone therapy on risk of hip and knee joint replacement in the Women's Health Initiative." *Arthritis Rheum* 54:3194-3204.

18. Cohen MS, Wall EJ, Kerber CW, et al. 1991. "The anatomy of the cauda equina on CT scans and MRI." *J Bone Joint Surg* 73-B:381-384.

19. Compagnone NA, Mellon SH,. 2000. "Neurosteroids: biosynthesis and function of these novel neuromodulators." *Front Neuroendocrinol* 21:1-56.

20. Coronel MF, Labomlorda F, Roig P, et al. 2011. "Progesterone prevents allodynia after experimental spinal cord injury." *J of Pain* 12:71-83.

21. Cutolo M. 2004. "Estrogen metabolites: increasing evidence for their role in rheumatoid arthritis and systemic lupus erythematosus." *J. Rheumatol* 31: 419–421.

22. Dahlhamer J, Lucas J, Zelaya C, et al. 2018. "Prevalence of chronic pain and high-impact chronic pain among adults." *United States, 2016 Mort & Mort Wkly Sept 14* 101-1006.

23. Damkier HH, Brown PD, Praetorius J,. 2013. "Cerebrospinal fluid secretion by the choroid plexus." *Physiol Rev* 93:1847-92.

24. Delamarter RB, Ross JS, Masaryk TS, etal. 1990. "Diagnosis of lumbar arachnoiditis by magnetic resonance imaging." *Spine* 15:304-310.

25. Deyo RA, Dvorkin SF, Antmann D, et al. 2014. "Report of the NIH Task Force on research standards for chronic low back pain." *J Pain* 115:569-585.

26. Deyo RA, Mirza Sk, Martin B,. 2006. "Back pain prevalence and visit rates: estimates from US Nation Surveys, 2002." *Spine* 31:2724-2727.

27. Djeball M, Guo Q, Pertus EH, et al. 2005. "The neurosteroids progesterone and allopregnanolone reduce cell death, gliosis, and functional deficits after traumatic brain injury in rats." *J Neurotrauma* 22:106-118.

28. Eisenberg E, Goldman R, Schlag-Eisenberg D, et al. 2019. "Adhesive arachnoiditis following lumbar epidural steroid injections: A report of two cases and review of literature." *J Pain Research* 12:513-518.

29. Elliott J. 1781. "Of the cure of sciatica in a complete collection of the medical and philosophical works of John Fothergill." p355-363. London: Pater-Nofter-Row.

30. Engstrand B, Carlstron K, Fellander-Tsai L, et al. 2003. "Abnormal levels of serum dehydroepiandrosterone, estrone, and estradiol in men with rheumatoid arthritis: high correlation between serum

estradiol and current degree of inflammation." *J. Rheumatol* 30: 2338-2343.

31. Epstein NE. 2013. "The risks of epidural and transforaminal steroid injections in the spine: commentary and a comprehensive review of the literature." *Surg Neurol* 4(supp2):574-593.

32. Evrard HC, Balthazart J,. 2004. "Rapid regulation of pain by estrogens synthesized in spinal dorsal horn neurons." *J Neurosci* 24:7225-7229.

33. Freburger JK, Holmes GM, Agans RP, et al. 2009. "The rising prevalence of chronic lower back pain." *Arch Intern Med* 169:251-258.

34. Freeman H, Pincus G, Bachrach S, et al. 1950. "Therapeutic efficacy of delta 5 pregnenolone in rheumatoid arthritis." *JAMA* 143:338-344.

35. Friedly J, Chan L, Deyo R,. 2007. "Increases in lumbosacral injections in the Medicare population." *Spine* 32:1754-1760.

36. Guth L, Zhang Z, Roberts E,. 1994. "Key role for pregnenolone in combination therapy that promotes recovery after spinal cord injury." *Proc Natl Acad Sci* 91:12308-12312.

37. Harbuz MS, Perveen-Gill Z, Lightman SL, et al. 1995. "A protective role for testosterone in adjuvant- induced arthritis." *Br J Rheumatol* 34:1117-1122.

38. Harrow T. 2018. "Epstein-Barr virus could be a cause of multiple autoimmune disorders." *VA Research Currents.* April 18.

39. Harvey SC. 1926. "Meningeal adhesions and their significance." *Interstate Post Grad Med, North America Prac* 2:27-31.

40. He J, Evans CO, Hoffman SW, et al. 2004. "Progesterone and allopregnanolone reduce inflammatory cytokines after traumatic brain injury." *Exp Neuro* 189:404-412.

41. Henderson FC, Austin C, Benzel E, et al. 2017. "Neurological and spinal manifestations of the Ehlers-Danlos Syndromes." *Amer J Men Gen* 175C:195-211.

42. Henschke N, Kamper SJ, Maher CG,. 2015. "The epidemiology and economic consequences of pain." *Mayo Clinic Proceeding* 90:139-147.

43. Hitt HC, McMillen RC, Thornton-Neurves T, et al. 2007. "Comorbidity of obesity and pain in a general population: results from the Southern Pain Prevalence Study." *J Pain* 8:430-436.

44. Homsi ME, Gharzeddine K, Cuevas J, et al. 2021. "MRI findings of arachnoiditis revisited: Is classification possible?" *J Morgan Rason Imaging* DOI:10.1002/jmri.27583.

45. Horsley V. 1909. "Chronic spinal meningitis: its differential diagnosis and surgical treatment." *Br J Med* 1:513-517.

46. Hoy D, March L, Brooks P, et al. 2014. "The global burden of low back pain: estimates from the Global Burden of Disease 2010 Study." *Ann Rheum Dis* 73:968-974.

47. Jackson A, Isherwood I,. 1994. "Does degenerative disease of the lumbar spine cause arachnoiditis? A magnetic resonance study and review of the literature." *Brit J Radiology* 67:840-847.

48. Javidi E, Magnus T,. 2019. "Autoimmunity after ischemic stroke and brain injury." *Fron in Immunol* 10:1.

49. Joels M, DeKloet E,. 1992. " Control of neuronal excitability by corticosteroid hormones." *Trends Neurosci* 15:25-30.

50. Jones KJ. 1993. "Gonadal steroids and neuronal regeneration: a therapeutic role." *Adv Neurol* 59:227-240.

51. Jorgenson J, Hansen PH, Steenskoo V, et al. 1975. "A clinical and radiological study of chronic lower spinal arachnoiditis." *Neuroradiology* 9:139-144.

52. Kalichman L, Cole R, Kim Dh, et al. 2009. "Spinal stenosis prevalence and association with symptoms: the Framingham Study." *Spine J* 9:545-550.

53. Katz JN, Harris MD. 2008. " Lumbar spinal stenosis." *N Engl J Med* 358:818-825.

54. Kennedy J, Roll JM, Schrauduer T, et al. 2014. "Prevalence of persistent pain in the US adult population: new data from the 2010 National Health Interview Survey." *J of Pain* 15:979-984.

55. Kiefer, etal. 1991. "Effects of dexamethasone on microglial activation in vitro." *J Neuroimmunology* 34:99-108.

56. Kiguch, et al. 2012. "Chemokines and cytokines in neuroinflammation leading to neuropathic pain." *Curr Opinion Pharmacol* 12:55-61.

57. Kiiski H, Aanismaa R, Tenhunen J, et al. s. 2013. "Healthy human CSF promotes glial differentiation of hESC-derived neural cells while retaining spontaneous activity in existing neuronal network." *Biology Open* 2:605-612.

58. Kilts JD, Tupler LA, Keefe FJ, et al. 2010. "Neurosteroids and self-reported pain in veterans who served in the Military after September 11,2001." *Pain Med* 10:1469-1476.

59. Kitson MC, Kostopanagiotau G, Alimeric K, et al. 2011. "Histopathological alterations after single epidural injection of rapivacaine, methylprednisolone acetate, or contrast material in swine." *Cardiovasc Intervert Radioil* 34:1288-1295.

60. Lei ZM, Rao CV. 2001. "Neural actions of luteinizing hormone and human chorionic gonadotropin." *Seminar Reprod Med* 19:103-109.

61. Loggia MI, Chunde DB, Oluwaseum A, et al. 2015. "Evidence for brain glial activation in chronic pain patients." *Brain* 138:604-615.

62. Manchikanti L, Singh V, Dalta S, et al. 2009. "Comprehensive Review of Epidemiology: scope and impact of spinal pain." *Pain Physician* 12:E35-E70.

63. McEwen BS, de Kloet ER, Rostene W. 1986. "Adrenal steroid receptors and action in the central nervous system." *Physio Rev* 66:1121-1188.

64. Meisel C, Schwab JM, Prass K, et al. 2005. "Central nervous system injury-induced immune deficiency syndrome." *Nat Rev Neurosci* 6:775-786.

65. Merck & Co. 1899. "Meningitis, Cerebral, Spinal, and Tubercular in Merck's 1899 Manual of the Materia Medica:." In *A Ready Reference Pocket Book for the Practicing Physician*, 146. New York: Merck & Co.

66. Mika J. 2008. "Modulation of microglia can attenuate neuropathic pain symptoms and enhance morphine effectiveness." *Pharmacol Rep* 60:297-300.

67. Murphy KR, Han JL, Yang S, et al. 2017. "Prevalence of specific types of pain diagnoses in a sample of United States adults." *Pain Phy* ;20:E257-E268.

68. Nahin RL. 2012. "Estimates of pain prevalence and severity in United States." *J Pain* 16:769-780.

69. Nelson DA. 1988. "Dangers from methylprednisolone acetate therapy by intraspinal injection." *Arch Neurol* 45:804-806.

70. O'Callgan JP, SriranT, Miller DB. 2008. "Defining "neuroinflammation."" *Ann NY Acad Sci* 1139:318-330.

71. Parenti V, Huda F, Richardson PK, et al. 2020. "Lumbar arachnoiditis: Does imaging associate with clinical features? ." *Clin Neurol Neurosurg* 192:105717.

72. Patil AA. 1990. "The effect of human chorionic gonadotropin (HCG) on restoration of the spinal cord: A preliminary report." *Int Surg* 75:54-57.

73. Patil AA, Nagaraj MP,. 1983. "The effect of human chorionic gonadotropin (HCG) on functional recovery of spinal cord sectioned rats." *ACTA Neurochir* 69:205-218.

74. Pitcher MH, von Koiff M, Bushnell CM, et al. 2019. "Prevalence and profile of high-impact chronic pain in the United States." *J Pain* 20:146-60,.

75. Quiles M, Marchiselo PJ, Tsairis P,. 1978. " Lumbar adhesive arachnoiditis: Etiologic and pathologic aspects." *Spine* 3:45-50.

76. Rajaee SS, Bae HW, Kanim LE, et al. 2012. "Spinal fusion in the United States: analysis of trends from 1998 to 2008." *Spine* 37:67-76.

77. Reddy DS. 2010. "Neurosteroids: endogenous role in the human brain and therapeutic potentials." *Prog Brain Res* 186:13-137.

78. Rodriguez LJG, Sandoval Sanchez V, Benavides Rodriguez D, et al. 2009. "Paraplegia due to adhesive arachnoiditis: a case report." *Act Ortop Mex* 23:232-236.

79. Roglio I, Bianchi R, Gotti S, et al. 2008. "Neuroprotective effects of dehydropresterone and progesterone in an experimental model of nerve crush injury." *Neurosci* 155:673-685.

80. Ross JS, Masaryk TS, Modic MT, et al. 1987. "MRI imaging of lumbar arachnoiditis ." *A J R Am J Roentgenol* ;149:1025-1032.

81. Rubin DI. 2007. "Epidemiology and risk factors for spine pain." *Neurol Clin* 25:353-371.

82. Schievink WI, Gordon OK, Tourje J, et al. 2004. "Connective tissue disorders with spontaneous spinal cerebrospinal fluid leaks and intracranial hypotension: a prospective study." *Neurosurgery* 54:65-71.

83. Sevesto S, Merli P, Ruggier M, et al. 2011. "Ehlers-Danlos Syndrome and neurological features: a review." *Childs Neuro Syst* 27:365-371.

84. Shealy CN. 1995. "A review of dehydroepiandrosterone (DHEA)." *Integ Physiol Behav Sci* ;30:308-313.

85. Shiraish T, Crook HV, Reynolds A. 1995. "Spinal arachnoiditis ossificans: Observations on its investigation and treatment." *European Spine J* 4:60-63.

86. Smith M, Davis MA, Stano M, et al. 2013. "Aging baby boomers and the rising cost of chronic back pain: secular trend analysis of longitudinal medical expenditures panel survey data for year 2000 to 2007." *J Manipulative Physiol Ther* 36:2-11.

87. Stookey B. 1927. "Adhesive spinal arachnoiditis simulating spinal cord tumor." *Arch Neurol and Psych* 17:151-164.

88. Strine TW, Hootman JM. 2007. "US national prevalence and correlation of low back and neck pain among adults." *Arthritis Rheum* 57:656-665.

89. Takahashi H, Suguro T, Okazima Y, etal. 1996. "Inflammatory cytokines in the herniated disc of the lumbar spine." *Spine* 21:218-224.

90. Takedo, etal. 2004. "Effect of methylprednisolone on neuropathic pain and spinal glial activation in rats." *Anesthesiology* 100:1249-1257.

91. Tennant F. 2016. "Arachnoiditis diagnosis and treatment." *Pract Pain Mgt* (14:63-69) 14:63-69.

92. Tennant F. 2009. "Human chorionic gonadotropin in pain treatment." *Prac Pain Mgt* 9:25-27.

93. Tennant F. 2013. "The physiologic effects of pain on the endocrine system." *Pain Ther* 2:75-86.

94. Tennant F. 2016. "Underlying causes of chronic pain which require high dose opioids. Pain Week (Las Vegas) and Amer Acad Pain Mgm (San Antonio)."

95. Tennant FS, Jr:. 1968. "The Glomerulonephritis of Infectious Mononucleosis." *Texas Reports on Biology and Medicine* 26:603-612.

96. Thomas J. 1873. "Arachnitis and Arachnoiditis." In *Comprehensive Medical Dictionary*, 57. Philadelphia: J.B. Lippincott & Co.

97. Thomson S. 2013. "Failed back surgery syndrome – definition, epidemiology, and demographics." *Br J Pain* 7:56-59.

98. Tsuda M. 2016. "Microglia in the spinal cord and neuropathic pain." *J Diabetes Investig* 7:17-26.

99. Wall, Chohen MS, Abithal JJ, et al. 1990. "Organization of intrathecal nerve roots at the level of conus medularis." *J Bone Joint Surg* ;72:1495-1499.

100. Wang L, Wang FS, Gershwin ME,. 2015. "Human autoimmune disease: a comprehensive update." *J Intern Med* 278:369-395.

101. Webster KM, Wright DK, Sun M, et al. 2015. "Progesterone treatment reduces neuroinflammation, oxidative stress and brain damage and improves long-term outcomes in a rat model of repeated mild traumatic brain injury." *J Neuroinflammation* 12:238.

102. Whendon JM, Glassey D,. 2009. "Cerebrospinal fluid stasis and its clinical significance." *Altern Ther Health Med* 15:54-60.

103. Yabuki S, Otqani K, Sekiguchii M, et al. 2013. "Prevalence of lumbar spinal stenosis using the diagnostic support tool, and correlated factors in Japan: a population-based study." *J Ortho Sci* 18:893-900.

104. Zang Y, Chee A, Shi P, etal. 2016. "Intervertebral disc cells produce interleukins found in patients with back pain." *Am J Phys Med* 95:407-415.

105. Zweiman B, Levinson AI,. 1992. "Immunologic aspects of neurological and neuromuscular diseases." *JAMA* 268:2918-2922.

INDEX

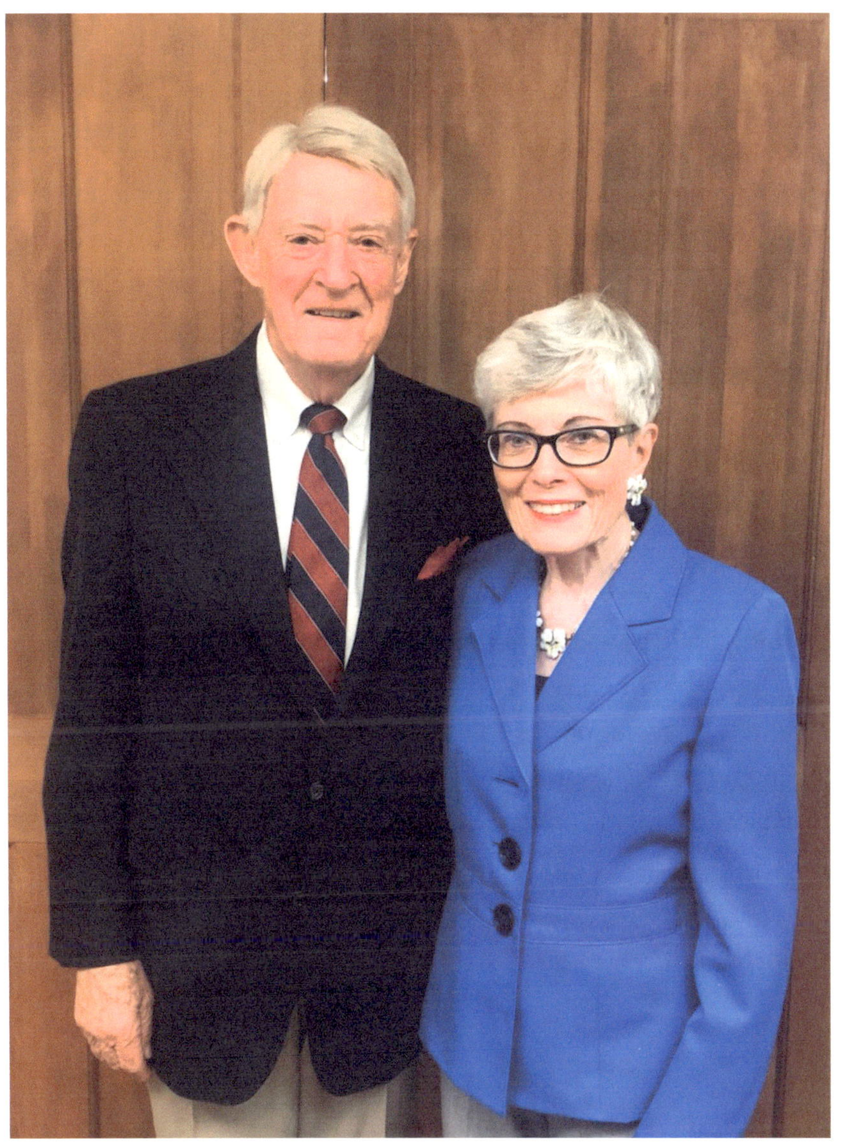

Forest and Miriam Tennant

ABOUT THE AUTHOR

Forest Tennant has spent most of his medical career as a practicing physician and researcher in the fields of addiction and pain medicine. He has published over 300 scientific articles and books in these fields. For his efforts he was given a "50 Year Achievement" award in 2017 by "Pain Week." In this 50-year span, he has been a US Army Medical Officer, UCLA Professor, Public Health Physician, and Drug Advisor for the Los Angeles Dodgers, NASCAR, and National Football League. He was editor of Practical Pain Management for 12 years. In 2018 he retired from clinical practice to do research on the spinal canal disease known as adhesive arachnoiditis. He and his wife, Miriam, have been married 55 years and they split their residence between West Covina, California and Wichita, Kansas, where they headquarter their real-estate company, Tennant Homes. Their charitable giving and medical research are sponsored by the Tennant Foundation.

OTHER BOOKS BY FOREST TENNANT

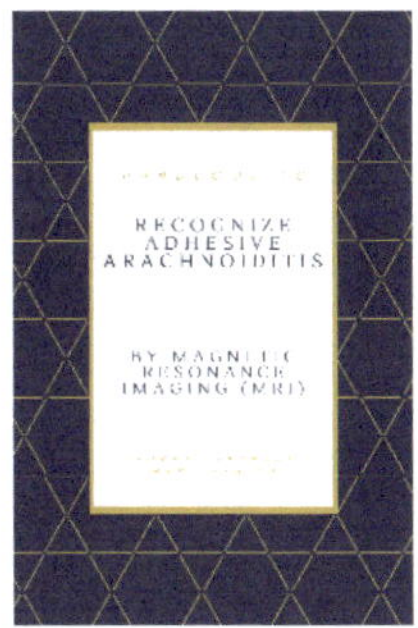

HANDBOOK TO RECOGNIZE ADHESIVE ARACHNOIDITIS BY MAGNETIC RESONANCE IMAGING (MRI)

ISBN:9781955934152
LOC: 2021925161

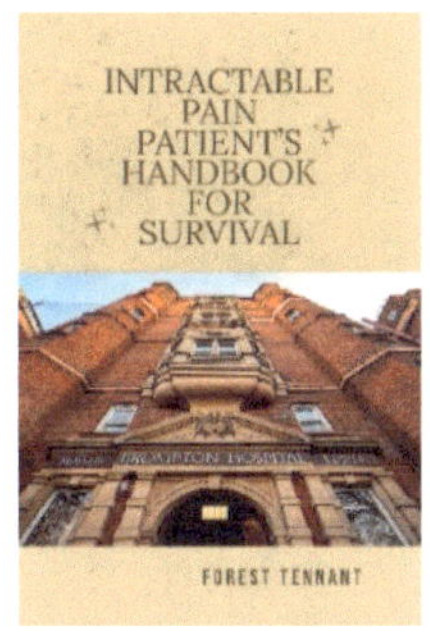

INTRACTABLE PAIN PATIENTS HANDBOOK FOR SURVIVAL

ISBN: 9781955934121
LOC: 2021916464

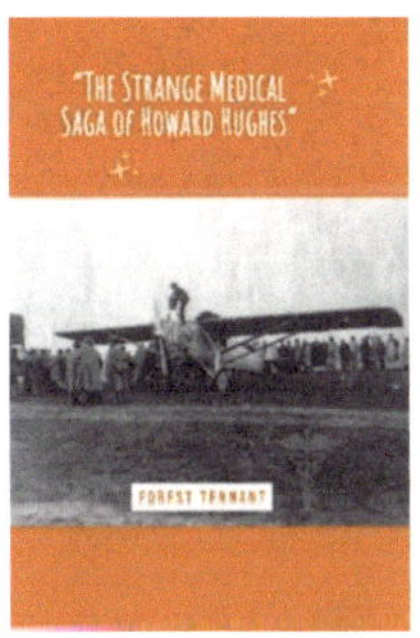

"THE STRANGE MEDICAL SAGA OF HOWARD HUGHES"

ISBN: 9781955934091
LOC: 2021912855

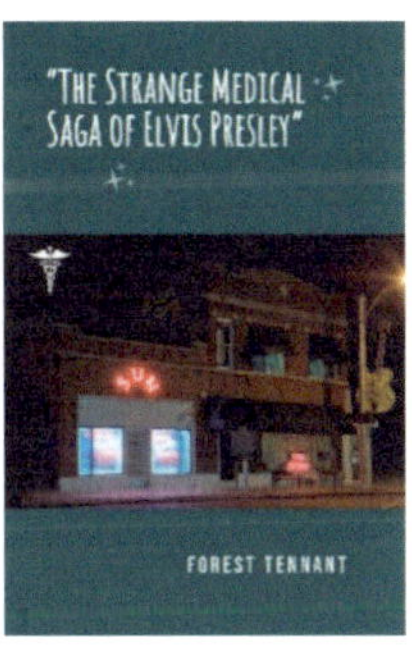

"THE STRANGE MEDICAL SAGA OF ELVIS PRESLEY"

ISBN: 9781955934008
LOC: 2021911718

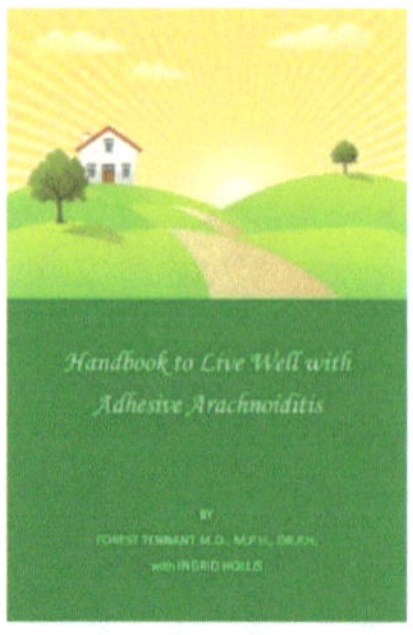

"HANDBOOK TO LIVE WELL WITH ADHESIVE ARACHNOIDITIS"

ISBN: 9781959340600
LOC: 2021912718

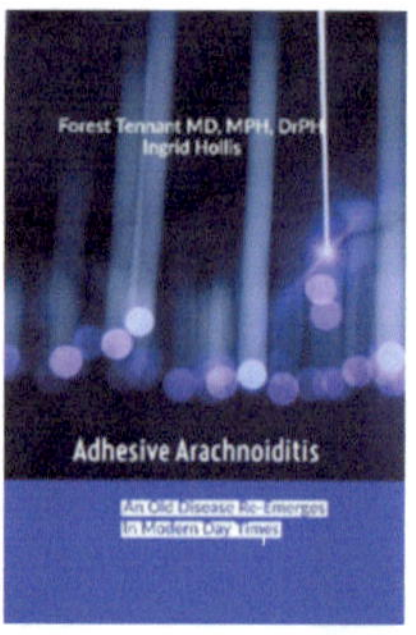

"ADHESIVE ARACHNOIDITIS: AN OLD DISEASE RE-EMERGES IN MODERN TIMES"

ISBN: 9781955934039
LOC:2021912467

Made in United States
Cleveland, OH
25 January 2025

13756071R10085